# The Black Woman's Guide to
# BEAUTIFUL HAIR

## A Positive Approach to Managing Any Hair Type and Style

**Lisa Akbari**

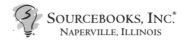

SOURCEBOOKS, INC.®
NAPERVILLE, ILLINOIS

Published by Sourcebooks, Inc.
P.O. Box 4410, Naperville, Illinois 60567-4410
(630) 961-3900
FAX: (630) 961-2168
www.sourcebooks.com

Library of Congress Cataloging-in-Publication Data

Akbari, Lisa.
        The black woman's guide to beautiful hair : a positive approach to managing any hair and style / Lisa Akbari.
              p.cm.
ISBN 1-57071-905-5 (alk. paper)
I. African American women—Health and hygiene. 2. Hair—Care and hygiene. 3. Beauty, Personal. I. Title.

RA778.4.A36 A337 2002
646.7'24'08996073—dc21

                                                                              2001057583

Printed and bound in the United States of America
BG   10  9  8  7  6  5  4  3

God blessed me with my hair, and God makes no mistakes.

# Acknowledgments

Heavenly, gracious, and merciful father, I thank you and give you all the praise and glory. Thank you for using me to be an answer to many prayers. God, I thank you for giving me the mind to ask questions, the determination to find the answer to the question, and the heart to want to share the answers with others. For this I am truly blessed and grateful.

To my husband Hooshang, thank you for being a true husband and a supportive friend.

Raumesh and Raumina, thank you for all the proofreading of my material, believing that I could do anything and for being the best daughters a mother could ever have.

To my mother, thank you for showing me that the world cannot stop me from doing anything, and if God is with me I can do all things.

To my agent Marlene Connor, thank you for saying to me that you believed that I was the one to write the hair book for black women and for never giving up on this book.

To my editor Deb Werksman, thank you for reading my material and believing that it is a good book.

And to the many clients who so graciously have expressed to me that they feel that I am a blessing to them. I would like to say to you that I feel blessed to have helped you to achieve your goals in obtaining healthy hair and healthy scalp.

# Table of Contents

# Introduction

The mission of this book is the same mission that I bring to my work with my individual clients—empowering you to embrace, respect, appreciate, and love your hair so that you will begin to care properly for and ultimately save your hair today, and for many years to come.

Now, let's be honest and admit that many of us from time to time say, "I really hate my hair." Some even say, "God was trying to punish black women when He gave us our hair." One of my eighty-year-old clients told me that it started way back when the pure black slave girls had true African kinky hair and the little mixed-

**You can learn to love your hair!**

breed sisters had that wavy hair. That is when we started believing that there was "good hair" and there was "bad hair." What a negative way to think about our hair!

Today there are many sisters who do not respect, appreciate, or understand their own hair in its natural state. Therefore, we abuse, misuse, bully, and try to change our hair in a misguided effort to control or manage it. We spend tons of money, time, and energy on weaving, waving, straightening, blow-drying, and curling, as we salon hop to find a way to have better hair. Then, we decide this is too much trouble and we cut our hair off and start over. No matter what we end up with, we still hate our hair. What gloom and doom!

Black women are caught between a rock and a hard place, confused and frustrated, wondering which way to go when it comes to our hair. So, what are you going to do? I will tell you what you are going to do. You are going to take charge. You are going to learn to love, appreciate, and care for your hair. Whether you start with natural hair or chemically treated hair, I am going to be right there with you and I will show you the way. If you have naturally kinky, dry hair, and you choose to chemically treat your hair, you will then have naturally kinky, dry, chemically treated hair. Underneath that change is still what was once kinky hair type and dry scalp. You must treat and care for it accordingly. No matter what you do to your hair, your hair and scalp will always require you to feed them what they naturally need and what they unnaturally need. Never forget that truth and you can stop some of your problems before they start.

This book will equip and empower you to succeed in having the kind of hair that you have dreamed of having, and thought you never could. What is better hair? Hair that is healthy, manageable, and loveable. You will be empowered to have better hair. I offer you a journey from unhealthy hair to healthy hair.

Together, we will go through cleansing and conditioning the hair, the mind, and the scalp. To cleanse is to remove the negative. In other words, stop doing and thinking things that cause damage or harm to your hair and scalp. To recondition is to replace the negative with the correct and positive. In other words, only think and do things that are healthy for your hair and scalp. In seven short weeks your mind, scalp, and hair will be cleansed and conditioned, creating an environment for healthy hair growth. To have better hair you'll start to build a strong foundation. That foundation is healthy, positive thoughts, a healthy scalp, and healthy hair.

First, you will learn exactly how to cleanse and condition the hair. We will learn about our hair, giving only the correct care to each and every strand, allowing all the strands to grow to their potential length and fullness. While you will now have a hair care regimen that will start you on your way, it is essential, and I urge you, to read this book in its entirety. If you do, you will have all the tools you need to make significant improvement in the quality of your hair in less than a two-month period.

You may start with your hair, but your success will depend on what's going on inside your mind. The second phase will be to cleanse and condition the mind. We will explore and expose the mind and its relationship to our hair. We will cleanse and recondition the mind

**Stop doing and thinking things that aren't the best for your hair and scalp.**

with positive thoughts about our hair, learn tools to shut out negativity about our hair, and begin to love our hair. As your attitude toward your hair improves, your hair will improve.

Then, we will cleanse and condition the scalp. Before healthy hair comes healthy scalp. Your scalp is the source of your beautiful hair. Therefore, we will prepare the scalp for hair growth, remove any blockage or negative buildup, cleanse the scalp, and prevent scalp damage. We will clear and heal the opening from which the hair extends, thus encouraging hair growth.

By the end of two months, if you've read this book and practiced what I'm recommending, you will have a head of better hair—not just temporarily, but for life!

## HEALTHY HAIR

Healthy hair for you may not be what you see on TV or in magazines. Healthy hair is hair that grows from a healthy scalp to its full potential length and fullness. When you complete this book, you will freely love your natural hair. If you choose to alter your hair in any way, you will be fully educated on your choices. You will know how to manage that choice and not let your choice manage you, and avoid hair and scalp problems. With all of our multiple hair textures and types we must be reminded of something very important. If you are black, you or someone in your family line has kinky hair and dry scalp. Hair and scalp problems will surface in some form if you deny this fact.

**Healthy hair, natural or styled!**

## MY STORY

About twenty-seven years ago, at age fifteen, I entered the hair care field. I was in the ninth grade in junior high school and my best friend was in the tenth grade in senior high school. One day, she took me to her cosmetology class, and I knew immediately that I wanted to be a hairstylist. The next year, I walked into that classroom and the same teacher, Mrs. Johnnie Brown, smiled as I filled out the enrollment card. I was there for the entire three-year course, and in 1977 I graduated from that cosmetology class with honors and also received my high school diploma.

The next month, I headed straight to the State Board and passed my board exams. I was officially a licensed cosmetologist. I felt truly blessed to know what I wanted to be at the very young age of seventeen. I opened my first full-service salon in 1981 at the age of twenty-one. This was a great time to be a hairstylist and salon life was very exciting. I felt that the time was a turning point in black hair care.

## A Good Turn That Went Bad

At that time, black women were getting tired of the "jheri curl" and were afraid to cut their hair. The "wrap" was still a thought to come. Sculptured hairstyles were getting harder and bigger. The professional and more conservative southern black female frowned and turned up her nose at any style that required the use of gel, grease, or curl activator. Black women seemed to have more pressure from their careers and jobs to look a certain way while still having a personal need to please their mates with their hairstyle choice. Many of my clients felt that they would have less style maintenance, and look more professional, with a short blow-dry and curl style, but did not think that their mates would be pleased.

One client really needed a neat, close-fitting professional hairstyle for her new job, and because she was pregnant, a low-maintenance style was a must. Yet, she did not want to ignore her husband's wishes that she not cut her hair. I had just completed a series of classes on "up styles," so I recommended a French roll style. That way she could have what she wanted, be in style, and please her husband. It was a solution that solved her problems and fit her lifestyle.

The French rolls and other low-maintenance styles were very popular with many black women. Some salons would advertise and compete for business, stating that their styles would hold longer than other salons. In my salon we called them sculpture styles. These styles would stay in place until shampooed out.

At the time I did not realize that this was a real turning point in black hair care—a bad turn. I went along with these creative money-making styles until clients went from keeping that style from week to week to two weeks or longer. One client actually went six full weeks. As the sculptures got bigger, many black women strayed away, wanting softer hairstyles. Blow-dry and curl styles and slick straight relaxers began to come into the picture. A new way to wave the hair then became popular. About 90 percent of my clients fluctuated between "soft styles" and "hard styles." They could not make up their minds. Half of the clients hated sculpture styles and half hated free-flowing styles. Both styles required the use of excessive heat or gel and harsh hairsprays. Blow-dry styles caused hair breakage and gel styles caused scalp problems. Most clients did not seem to mind and complained very little, thinking it was just the price they had to pay in order to be beautiful.

When the wrap became popular, hairstylists thought they were saved because this style seemed to satisfy almost every client. The wrap offered a low-maintenance style that our sculpture clients wanted, and then it also offered a free-flowing style, with the body and bounce our blow-dry and curl clients wanted, without the itch, flaky scalp, and hair breakage. When the client came out from under the dryer and the hair was unwrapped, it would fall into place. What I liked most about the wrap was that there was no need for gel, harsh sprays, or excessive heat, and clients' hair seemed to grow faster. The hair and scalp seemed to be in better condition. Unfortunately, then we started using the flat iron, a metal tool with a handle like a curling iron and an end shaped like a duck's beak. This tool was used to give the wrap more shape, but instead it eventually burned the hair.

> **Both "soft styles" and "hard styles" require the use of excessive heat or harsh products.**

## Trouble on the Horizon

I could see the slow rise of hair and scalp problems among black women as the demands for just the right hairstyle or look became an obsession. We found a way to damage our hair even with the wrap. Many clients ran back to press and curl hair, but found that it was no longer a solution. Black women had become obsessed with straight hair. I call it the era of "relaxer addiction." We did not want to admit it then because we were afraid it would be misinterpreted. It was not because we wanted to be like our white sisters. No, we are and always have been proud of our ethnicity.

I believe, and I am speaking as a black women as well as a stylist who saw her clients go through this, that we were simply trying

**Hair and scalp problems among black women are on the rise.**

to find a way to manage our hair with the least maintenance possible. Straighter hair seems to do that for us. Systematically, the media and advertisements portray straight hair as the only really beautiful hair. Opportunists make big profits from selling relaxers not only to salons, but over the counter. Black women and men have become brainwashed and, as a race of people, have never learned how to take care of and manage their natural kinky hair. Therefore, we never learned to love and appreciate our hair before we altered it.

By 1985, after being a stylist for almost a decade and a salon owner for almost five years, I became depressed and fed up with salon life. To most I was a rising star stylist. I could cut, curl, and style in fifteen minutes—and put together a French roll in less than ten minutes. At the peak of my career as a stylist, I averaged $3,500 a week, had five personal assistants, and a line of clients waiting to get into my chair. Yet something was wrong. I was no longer happy as a stylist. I was torn because I loved my clients and I really loved doing hair. I even expanded my fourteen hundred square foot hair salon into a thirty-eight hundred square foot day spa, adding a nail salon, tanning bed, boutique, skin care, massage, whirlpool, sauna, fully equipped workout gym, juice bar, and limousine service. This new "salon plus" was the talk of the town, and was the largest full-service salon in Memphis and in the state of Tennessee. I received a two-page write-up in *Shop Talk* magazine. This was all very nice and very grand, but I still felt something was missing. I was in a rut. Somehow, I was off track.

I had become a stylist in order to make a difference. In my early years as a student and then stylist, I did see some flaky scalps and hair breakage, but nothing like what was beginning to happen. Black women were losing hair and their scalp problems were increasing at an alarming rate. Only a small percentage of black women had healthy hair. The problem stemmed from poor scalp and hair care habits, and an attitude from stylists as well as clients to get the style at whatever cost. Hair care professionals styled hair with little or no consideration for the hair or scalp. We thought that this was what had to be done in order to get the "look." Beauty schools were no better—they had no curricula that adequately addressed the hair and scalp problems black women face when trying to manage and style their hair. What hope did we have for the future stylist?

**Only a small percentage of black women have healthy hair, but now you can be one of them.**

Although my clients had pretty haircuts and styles, their hair and scalp did not seem as healthy as I thought it could be. The products and education available did not address both style and care. There had to be a way for black women to have any hairstyle they wanted and still have healthy hair and a healthy scalp.

### Taking Charge

To find a solution, I enrolled in advanced hair classes and product knowledge classes held by manufacturers. My goal was to learn as much as possible about the hair, scalp care, and available styling products. I was looking for styling techniques and products that would allow me to protect, preserve, and care for my clients' hair while achieving the desired style. Because I had such expert styling skills, I even became a platform artist for one company. While their sales went through the roof, I knew in my heart that their product did not address any of the hair and scalp problems that black women were facing.

I wanted to work for a manufacturer that would educate me on styling with products while protecting and preserving the hair. I never found the right one. Although many manufacturers had the money and resources to find the answers, most were playing copycat with each other and some just covered up the problems. Many had one or two products in their line that came close to giving some relief, but without a complete system and no real education for the professional as well as the consumer, these products never seemed to quite get to the root of the problem.

Ultimately, all my help came from God. I prayed to my heavenly Father for guidance and he directed me to answers. It was like being back in school. I started to really study, test, and research. I studied all textures and types of hair strands, tested chemicals, shampoos, conditioners, moisturizers, oils, grease products, gels, setting lotions, hairsprays, and heat styling tools to see the different effects that each had on kinky hair and dry scalp. I read every book in my local library on the skin and on hair loss that was written by a dermatologist. I spent hours in the medical library looking for research on hair and scalp problems of blacks.

My research answered many questions for me about why many black women suffered with hair and scalp problems. I found that the reason for the phenomenon was that we were overlooking one very important fact, and paying for it dearly. My black clients with kinky hair type and dry scalp had different needs than my white clients with straight hair type and oily scalp. Obviously, it does not take a rocket scientist to see this, but even though we knew there was a difference, we did nothing about it. The beauty schools grouped blacks and whites together, using the same products and styling techniques on both. Manufacturers supposedly produced hair products made for black hair care, but hadn't really taken the time to study kinky hair and dry scalp. We needed products that were more than just an afterthought.

**Kinky hair type and dry scalp have different needs than straight hair type and oily scalp.**

When we stood over the clients' heads and saw how hair strands began to thin, short hair spots began to appear, and the scalp began to deteriorate, we never said a word; we just styled it differently so the client would not notice. When the problem got so bad and the client said something to us, we said it must be stress, nerves, or age. We suggested weaves, which only covered up the problem or made it worse. If that client pushed the issue of her hair and scalp problems, some of us would avoid her or take her off our book, labeling that client as a picky problem client, making her think it was something she must be doing wrong at home. Some stylists only wanted to work on perfect heads, without accepting the fact that they were responsible for many of the hair and scalp problems. Many clients would just sit in a stylist's chair, week after week for years, until they were literally bald, trusting and thinking that if she just hung in there, it would get better and her hair would one day be the way it had been when she first started coming to that stylist. Needless to say, it didn't usually happen.

## WHAT IS GOING ON WITH HAIR CARE

Products and hair care programs are not protecting and preserving black hair and scalp. The styling products and techniques we are using are causing damage to our hair. Many of my colleagues in the hair care profession will argue that hair is hair and it is all the same. I strongly disagree. Although hair strands have three

**Black women can learn to know their hair.**

basic layers made of protein, cells, and fiber, kinky hair and straight hair are not the same. Kinky hair is not only structurally different, but also needs different hair and scalp styling and maintenance than straight hair does. Historically, we have let other races of people tell us what to do, including how to care for our hair. Also, many black women are not aware of the negative and incorrect thoughts and habits that control how they view and deal with their hair and scalp.

In my interviews with women who have hair problems, I hear a lot of excuses for why they cannot seem to change their bad habits. We put everything and everybody in front of hair care. The truth of the matter is that black women have never put as much attention on hair care as they put on hairstyles or how our hair looks. We have not been taught the importance of good scalp and hair cleaning and conditioning. As a race, we have not come to know our hair. And the problem is getting worse.

One evening after doing my round-table live TV talk show, some of the guests on my show told me how much they enjoyed the show and how important a show like this one was to black women. I will never forget something that one of my guests said to me: "You know, Mrs. Akbari, we have a generation that does not know what their natural hair looks like." She was right. Each year I treat hundreds of children under age ten for scalp and hair damage because of chemical relaxers. These are children whose moms put relaxer in their hair as early as two years old. I have found that the younger the mom, the younger the child was when she received her first relaxer. So-called "kiddy perms" are now available under everybody's hair label. This is one of the fastest-growing products in the relaxer market, now outselling the so-called "no lye" relaxers. Somehow, manufacturers have convinced moms across the country that these "kiddy perms" are mild and won't hurt a child's hair. Moms are not only using them on their girls' hair, but because they are convinced that they are so mild, they are now using them on their own hair. But, a chemical is a chemical, and all chemicals have the potential to do harm to the hair and scalp.

## THE ANSWER

After many years, thousands of interviews, and countless hours of testing and studying the hair and scalp of black women, I realized that more than 90 percent of my clients were suffering from the same problems. Although they came from different sources, the problems were the same: dry scalp and weak hair. I knew that if I could get my clients to understand the differences of black hair and scalp, I could teach them how to have better hair.

First, I had my clients come in for a consultation and hair analysis to determine the problem and treatment. Each client is taught to be proud of the hair God blessed her with. Then, they learn about scalp and hair type. After the initial consultation, the client is put on a program of hair and scalp treatments. By treating the hair and scalp in the correct way, I create an environment for healthy hair growth. I discovered that after the first treatment the hair and scalp look and feel better. In four weeks of treatment, clients who suffered with dry, tight, itchy, or flaky scalp reported that the problem was completely gone.

**Once you understand what your hair needs, you can have better hair.**

The condition of the hair improves dramatically as well. In seven weeks all my clients who stay with the treatment program report that their hair and scalp have never been in such great condition. Their hair strands have more elasticity, as well as equal porosity, meaning the ability to absorb hair products and chemicals in a controlled manner. The new growth has true texture, and the natural kinky hair type is extremely manageable. Many clients with scalp disorders have told me that their dermatologists say that whatever they are doing is working and to keep doing it. I began to praise my Heavenly Father for using me as a tool to bring this to black women.

The seven-week program will give you a foundation to build healthy hair now, and in years to come. This book is not about blaming any other group of people for the hair and scalp problems that plague black women. It is about taking care of ourselves and becoming empowered to help ourselves. You do not have to give up your favorite style choices in order to build a good foundation and find your way home to better hair. You just need new tools and a new road map.

In this program, I will not tell you if you should wear your hair natural or chemically straightened. That is, and should always be, your choice. However, I warn you that you cannot

**This book will give you easy steps to proper scalp and hair care, no matter what your choice of style is.**

and should not become solely dependent upon chemicals and pressing to give you better hair. Consider forms of straightening processes only to assist in manageability and the style versatility of your hair. Straightening processes are only options in managing and styling kinky hair type, and are not the way to healthy hair. Also, you will not want to become chemical dependent, or over use straightening processes, resulting in damage to your hair and scalp.

This book will give you very easy steps on proper scalp and hair care, no matter what your choice of style is.

# *The Program*

You are about to embark on a simple program that you must do continuously for a period of seven weeks. If you do, your hair will be yours to manage, love, and care for as the crowning glory it is, for the rest of your days. I believe that in order to have better hair and scalp you must have a program that works with your hair and scalp type, not against it. This program will work for all different types of hair and scalp, including yours!

## FIRST STEP: CLEAN HOUSE

Start by going in your bathroom, dresser, under your cabinet, or wherever you keep your hair and scalp care products. Now take them all out and sit them on your dining room table. Get a pen and pad, and write down the name of each product, making columns beside each one. This is going to be called your product evaluation sheet.

If you are happy and your hair and scalp are healthy, then go ahead and use the products you already have in your seven-week program. If not, stay tuned—I have some suggestions. Throw away the products that don't pass evaluation.

| Name of Product | pH of Shampoo | Yes/No |
|---|---|---|
| *Shampoo* | | |
| • Do my scalp and hair feel clean? | | |
| • Does my hair feel dry? | | |
| • Does my hair feel soft? | | |
| • Does my hair feel strong? | | |
| • Does my hair break? | | |
| • Does my scalp feel better than it did before I used the product? | | |
| • Does my scalp itch? | | |
| • Does my hair shine? | | |
| • Does my hair look dull? | | |
| • Does my style hold without damage? | | |
| *Oil/Moisturizer* | | |
| • Do my scalp and hair feel clean? | | |
| • Does my hair feel dry? | | |
| • Does my hair feel soft? | | |
| • Does my hair feel strong? | | |
| • Does my hair break? | | |
| • Does my scalp feel better than it did before I used the product? | | |
| • Does my scalp itch? | | |

| Name of Product | pH of Shampoo | Yes/No |
|---|---|---|
| • Does my hair shine? | | |
| • Does my hair look dull? | | |
| • Does my style hold without damage? | | |
| *Conditioner* | | |
| • Do my scalp and hair feel clean? | | |
| • Does my hair feel dry? | | |
| • Does my hair feel soft? | | |
| • Does my hair feel strong? | | |
| • Does my hair break? | | |
| • Does my scalp feel better than it did before I used the product? | | |
| • Does my scalp itch? | | |
| • Does my hair shine? | | |
| • Does my hair look dull? | | |
| • Does my style hold without damage? | | |

## SECOND STEP: HOME HAIR AND SCALP CARE KIT

In order to have a successful program you will need the proper tools. Right now you must put together a home hair care maintenance kit. The size of the kit will depend on how versatile you wish to be with your hairstyles—a small piece of luggage should be

**Throw away any products that aren't up to standard.**

fine. Putting together a kit is a necessity. How many times have you gone crazy because your two-year-old thought your roller was a toy, or you just misplaced those clips? Keeping things together will help.

### Sample Kit for Natural Kinky Hair Type

- Large-tooth combs, butterfly clips, satin ponytail holders, and Zip-lock baggies to keep small items together.
- Plastic caps and a table-top dryer—for deep conditioning.
- A date book to keep track of salon visits.
- Shampoo, conditioner, leave-in conditioner, oil, and a moisturizer.

### Sample Kit for Chemically Treated Kinky Hair Type

- Large- and small-tooth combs as well as rattail combs for setting the hair.
- Hair rollers and rods, butterfly clips, roller clips, end wraps, and Zip-lock baggies to keep small items together.
- Plastic caps and a table-top dryer—for deep conditioning.
- A date book to keep track of chemical services and salon visits.
- Shampoo, conditioner, leave-in conditioner, oil, and a moisturizer.
- A sculptor setting tool, and a sculptor misting holding spray.

## THIRD STEP: CLEANSING, CONDITIONING, STYLE, AND SUPPORT

You should always look at three main areas of your hair and scalp regimen: cleansing, conditioning, and styling. You should also learn how to support your hair during these processes. Cleansing includes creating an environment for hair growth, removing all mental negatives, and letting the healing take place. Your goal is to create an environment for healthy hair growth. You will remove all negative buildups from the hair and scalp, allowing the

**Cleansing creates an environment for healing.**

healing and cleansing process to begin. You will then start your deep reconditioning process. All of this will allow your hair to grow to its potential length and fullness, becoming as long and as full as you desire.

## CLEANSE

To begin, focus on clarifying first the scalp and then the hair. Clarifying means to remove all unnatural things from the surface of the hair and scalp, placing it in a pure, clean state. Clarifying does not mean to strip. Stripping the hair and scalp will not only remove unnatural things

**pH of 4.5 to 5.5 is healthy for your hair. Never go over pH 6 in any shampoo.**

from the hair, but will also cause the hair and scalp to become dry because stripping removes any trace of natural oils and moisture. I recommend that you use a cleaning, clarifying, and acid-balanced shampoo with a pH of 5.5.

### The right shampoo

Always use the proper shampoo, one that is the pH of your hair and scalp. Many may think that all shampoos are the same, but that is simply not true. Some shampoos can cause a negative buildup or cause your scalp to dry out. And many shampoos on the market today have a very high pH.

Your scalp and hair have a pH of 4.5 to 5.5. In order to have a healthy scalp and encourage hair growth, stay as close to the natural pH as possible. Never go past pH 6.

Never use all-in-one shampoos. Some shampoos claim to clean and condition hair at the same time. These shampoos never get the scalp clean and cause a flaky buildup on the hair and scalp, which at some point could lead to low- and even high-level scalp damage.

### Shampoo in the shower

In the clarifying process, you also will need a large supply of very warm, forceful water, not just running water. I recommend that you shampoo in the shower using a handheld shower attachment. Do not put your head under the sink or tub.

My studies have shown that you will do a better job shampooing your hair and scalp in the shower and you will have fewer scalp problems. Being in the shower allows for a better water force, better cleansing, and saved time. If you hold your head over a sink, you will not be able to rinse the back of the neck area well, nor will you be able to rinse the front of your head properly, no matter how hard you try.

**Leaning over the sink, you won't be able to rinse properly. Get in the shower!**

Check your showerhead and make sure that you have a dial massager, the kind that changes from one type of force to another.

(A handheld showerhead will make rinses easier, but is not necessary.) You can adjust the dial massager for mild pressure for a sensitive or damaged scalp, and as the scalp heals you can change the dial for a deeper scalp massage.

### Steps for cleansing

Before you shampoo, slide your fingers through your hair, gently removing any tangles. (There is no need to brush or comb your hair.)

There is a correct way and an incorrect way to shampoo your hair. Each time you shampoo your hair, plan to apply shampoo twice: prerinse scalp and hair, shampoo, rinse, and repeat shampoo and rinse.

### Prerinsing Scalp & Hair

Rinsing well *before* you apply shampoo is very important. It removes all of the immediate topical things like dust, lint, and other debris that are just sitting on the hair and scalp surface. Prerinsing may take from sixty seconds to three minutes. It is important to follow these simple, quick steps and not to rush.

Start by rinsing your scalp, making small openings or parts in your hair with your fingers while aiming warm, forceful water directly onto the scalp. Focus on scalp areas in the crown, the nape, behind the ears, and the hairline. Proper scalp rinsing is very important in cases where scalp itch and flakes are present. In cases involving scalp problems, rinse with almost-hot water (be careful that it's not too hot) directly into itchy, flaky areas for an extra sixty seconds.

Next, rinse your hair by slighting tilting your head forward, allowing the hair to fall forward on each side of the head, almost creating a part straight down the back of the head. Allow the water to flow through the hair as you slide your fingers gently through your hair strands. This is a very important step in proper rinsing of long hair because it prevents tangles.

### Shampooing Scalp and Hair

Never dump the shampoo on your head. Instead, pour it into your hands and rub your palms together, spreading the shampoo down your fingers. Next, make small parts and openings in the hair and apply shampoo to your scalp with the same focus on areas of the scalp that you had during prerinsing. Apply shampoo to your scalp quickly in large sections. Slide or rub your fingers through the hair, allowing shampoo to move toward strand ends.

Never massage on top of your hair—slide your fingers under your hair directly on your scalp, then slide your fingers through to the ends. This will prevent matting, tangles, and damage to the hair shaft. Use the balls of the fingers on both hands to massage the scalp, and use your forefingers (not your fingernails) to gently massage shampoo into dry, flaky, or itchy spots. Never use your fingernails or any sharp objects, as these will cause scalp damage.

### Rinse and repeat

After your first shampoo, rinse your hair and scalp as described above for one or two minutes, then reapply shampoo as described above.

### Check to be sure your scalp is clean

Take a white hand towel and wrap the corner around your forefinger, gently rubbing your scalp in different areas, focusing on the scalp areas that may have itched. Look at the towel—if it is brown or discolored in any way, then your scalp is not clean or properly rinsed. Repeat the step on scalp rinsing and do the towel test again. If necessary, repeat the scalp-shampoo and scalp-rinsing steps. Now, feel your scalp and hair—they should be squeaky clean.

Do not be alarmed if your hair feels dry after the hair shampooing steps. You may only notice this happening the first week, but it may last for the first four weeks, depending on how low the moisture level of your damaged hair is. As long as your shampoo is pH 5.5, then the dryness is only from all of the negative buildup being removed. Remember, the clarifying process will remove all unnatural things from the hair strands, and that includes hair products that you have used in the past that may have made your hair soft but were not treating and improving the condition of your hair, only covering up your hair problem. By the time you finish the reconditioning steps, your protein and moisture levels will be balanced and your hair will not only feel great, but it will be in better condition.

**Make sure your scalp is clean before you condition.**

## CONDITION

Proper conditioning is very important, and there is a correct way to condition your hair. Here are instructions to follow if your hair is not damaged. If your hair is damaged, you should then go on to the section on reconditioning.

After shampooing, towel-dry your hair in order to remove excess water. It is important to remove as much water as possible so that your conditioner will attach to the hair surface and will not be diluted or roll off with the water. Removing the excess water will allow your conditioner to have more direct contact with your hair strands. To towel-dry your hair, place a large towel over your head and open the hair, gently blotting the hair closest to the scalp first, then blotting and squeezing all the strands to the ends. Never handle your hair in a rough manner. Another way to remove the excess water is to wrap your hair with a towel and leave it there for five minutes.

**Towel-dry first to allow conditioner to attach to the hair surface.**

Make openings and parts in your hair, then apply conditioner with your fingers so that you can place the conditioner onto the hair closest to your scalp. Next, apply conditioner to the ends of the hair. Then apply to the entire strand. If the hair has tangles, apply extra conditioner directly onto the tangled areas, then use your forefinger and thumb to massage tangles away. Do not comb conditioner through, as this will cause too much strain on the strands. Allow the conditioner to work first.

**Combing conditioner through strains your strands. Just let it sit.**

When conditioning long hair, apply conditioner to your hands, then rub it into your hair starting at the ends and working up to the scalp area. Next, slide your fingers throughout all the strands for even distribution.

Depending on the condition of your hair, you can now rinse the conditioner out thoroughly, or deep condition by keeping it on under the dryer for a few minutes as described in the next section.

## HAIR REPAIR

Proper conditioning of the hair is very important. When hair becomes damaged, thin, and breaks, there is no way to completely repair the damaged hair strand. You will never be able to reattach the lost cuticle layers that caused the strand thinning or put back the lost strands that broke off and caused short, weak spots to appear. But, this reconditioning program will empower you to protect and preserve the damaged layers and strands by raising and balancing the moisture and protein levels of the strands. This will soften and strengthen the hair. This will also increase the elasticity of the strands so that the hair does not break. Also, the cuticle layers of your hair strands will become more compact and will not peel. The strand-thinning process will stop. This program will not bring your damaged hair back to its original natural state—nothing will do that—but you will recondition it and have better hair.

You have two options for dealing with damaged hair: you can choose to cut it off, or you can choose to treat and recondition the damaged strands. It is important that you make a choice, and it is also important that, **Baby your hair strands.** when you make your choice, you are ready to live with it. In other words, if you cut your damaged strands off and start over, and if you have put much thought in this decision, then it is OK. If you choose to treat and recondition your hair, then you must understand you also have chosen to deal with or baby your damaged strands. As long as it is your well-thought-out choice, then that is OK. I want you to understand that this choice to recondition your damaged strands will mean that you must be very careful in every step of how you handle your hair.

Most women choose to keep their long hair and recondition it rather than cut it off. You may have some ups and downs during this process, but you will be empowered to have better hair. Stay focused, pay close attention to my instructions, don't let fear in, and you will do just fine. Whether your hair is breaking a little or a lot, you can follow this program and have better hair. Remember that your damaged hair strands are a part of you that has become weak and is in need of some tender loving care. You will baby your hair back to health.

## Reconditioning

In order to have true, deep reconditioning of the damaged strands, you must have maximum penetration of your conditioner into the cuticle layers of your hair strands. To achieve this, I recommend that you use a deep-penetrating, protein-and-moisture-rich conditioner in order to stabilize the hair strands, and use the following method.

After shampooing, towel-dry your hair and apply conditioner as described earlier. Then, using both hands, gently rub all your hair toward the crown of your head and cover it with a plastic cap. Sit under a warm dryer for fifteen minutes (the dryer should be set on medium). Come out from under the dryer, remove the cap, and carefully apply more conditioner to the hairline, to the ends, and to any short, weak spots, as well as to any areas where strand thinning has occurred. Cover with a cap as before and sit back under the dryer for ten more minutes. Come out from under the dryer and again apply additional conditioner to hairline, ends, and weak spots. Cover with a cap and sit back under the dryer for another ten minutes, for a total of thirty-five minutes. Finally, rinse your hair thoroughly for at least sixty seconds.

**Protect your hair with leave-in conditioner.**

### Leave-in conditioner

Whether your hair is damaged or just kinky, it is important to protect it. A leave-in conditioner will add elasticity to your strands by placing a positive buildup on the hair shaft, and will protect your hair from styling and everyday handling. For damaged hair, the protective buildup of a leave-in conditioner is like a cast to a broken bone or bandage to a wound—it protects the strands as they recondition. Use a lightweight leave-in conditioner (such as Hair Vitamin leave-in conditioner) that is water-soluble and will rinse clean from the strands as soon as warm water is applied.

**Always work tangles out before combing.**

Towel-blot in a squeezing motion to remove excess water (remember, too much water dilutes conditioner). Spray on leave-in conditioner, taking care to get inside any new growth and the hair closest to the scalp and onto the ends, then massage in. If there are any tangles, use your thumb and forefinger to massage the leave-in directly into the tangled areas. Next, finger-comb your hair; then, using a large, wide-tooth comb, gently comb through your hair. Remember, never comb before tangles are removed.

## COMBING AND BRUSHING
### Proper combing

Combing your hair in a gentle, loving way is very important in preserving the cuticle layers. Always use a comb that is appropriate for your hair length, texture, and type. The longer your hair is, the larger your comb should be, and the shorter your hair is, the smaller your comb should be. Fine hair strands are smaller, so it is very important that you use a large comb with teeth widely spread apart for less stress on the strands. Take into consideration whether you have natural or chemically treated hair. With natural hair, no matter what texture or length, you must use a large, wide-tooth comb to prevent excess pulling.

A leave-in conditioner can make combing easier. Finger massage your leave-in conditioner into tangled areas and into your entire head of hair. Be sure that your fingers flow smoothly through before placing a comb in your hair. Apply more leave-in

**Brushing can scratch your scalp and tear your hair.**

moisturizer for natural hair, or, for chemically treated hair, apply leave-in hair vitamins. As your hair gets into better condition, you will notice fewer problems with tangles. You may comb your hair from scalp area to ends, but the second you get to a matted or tangled area, you must go to the ends and comb from the ends, working back toward the tangled area, carefully combing in a raking motion. It is like removing a knot out of thread. Remember to apply more leave-in conditioner directly into tangles and finger massage as needed.

## Brushing

Down through the years, from one generation to the next, women have been told that they should brush their hair. A survey that I conducted revealed that many women thought that brushing would somehow give them better hair. Brushing the scalp stimulates circulation and may in some cases have positive effects on the scalp, causing the scalp to become more relaxed. On the other hand, brushing the scalp and hair can be very dangerous and damaging when nylon or pointed-bristle brushes are used. These types of brushes will scratch the scalp and tear the hair cuticles. Then, as you have learned, the scalp immediately goes into a self-healing mode and itches, becomes tight, tender, and dry. The hair cuticles will become torn and weak, causing hair frizzing and poor elasticity.

**Your hairstyle is up to you, but use products and techniques that won't hurt your hair.**

If you feel the need to brush your hair, I recommend that you only use a brush with straight plastic bristles that have a small round ball on the tip of each bristle. This type of brush will give some style benefits as well as relaxation to the scalp.

## SUPPORT PRODUCTS

This part of the program is to be used as needed to give your hair added softness and shine, as well as better style retention. Support products also can help relieve a dry scalp. Remember, the support program can and should be used with the reconditioning as well as the style aspects of your program.

Two products I recommend are Moisture Plus Moisturizer and Oil Sheen in a Jar. Below I have listed some ways to use these support products. Use support products as needed, keeping in mind this rule of thumb: moisturizer is needed when the hair feels dry or the scalp feels tight, and oil is needed when the hair looks dull or the scalp is dry or flaky.

### Moisturizer

Naturally, you will use moisturizer on your hair if it feels dry. Also use it on natural hair or new growth for softness and manageability. Use moisturizer on wet hair to hold or retain moisture in the hair, and on dry hair to raise the moisture level in the hair. Be sure to allow a moisturizer to dry in your hair before using a press. Use around your hairline to lay it down to replace gel.

### Oil

If your hair looks dry, oil can be used to improve luster. It can be used on color-treated hair. Use it on hair ends to seal split ends. Use oil on your scalp only during the dry-scalp phase of healing, or if you wear any style that is confined or close fitting to your head.

## STYLE GUIDE

Styling is an area where many women get themselves into trouble. Your choice of style isn't the problem—it's the products and techniques, such as gel, spritz, grease, or crimping with a too-hot crimping iron, etc. In the past, many of you have used damaging styling products and have worn styles that caused damage to your hair and scalp. But that is about to change.

This part of your program is very important because you do not want to undo all your efforts to recondition with poor styling habits, bad products, and negative actions. Don't forget that care comes before style. I define negative as wrong, incorrect, out of order, destructive, or with potential for harm. I don't particularly recommend heated styling tools, but if you choose to style using them then you must use with care.

### Roller Set (Wet Setting)

Roller setting the hair is the safest way to style. First shampoo, condition, and remove excess water from the hair, then apply a "Sculptor Set" to your strands. Avoid gel, which will dry your scalp and hair and cause negative buildup, and mousse, which will cause your strands to puff up and dry out. Now, choose magnetic smooth rollers in the size you prefer and roll them carefully into your hair.

I recommend a tabletop hard-head type hair dryer, rather than a bonnet type, which tends to be too confining to the head and will overheat the scalp and dry out the hair. Set the dryer on the medium setting. Turn the dryer on when you are ready to sit under it, so your scalp will warm up as the dryer does. This is even more important if you have scalp problems.

Sipping cool water while under the dryer will keep your body temperature normal and prevent sweating.

Remember that most of the dryer heat is directed to the crown of your head, so apply a small amount of moisturizer on the hair and scalp in the crown area a few times as the hair dries.

After you have sat under the dryer for a few minutes, be sure to rotate each roller. Place your forefinger and thumb on the end of the roller, press the roller down gently, then turn it in the opposite direction to the way it is turned in your hair. This allows the ends of the hair to dry faster and will cut your dryer time in half.

## Heated styling tools

I believe that heated styling tools are the second leading cause of hair loss among women, chemicals being number one. The use of heated styling tools is a case of a good thing gone bad. You can use heated styling tools such as a blow-dryer, curling iron, pressing comb, and even hot rollers without hair loss, if used in correct moderation. But this is direct heat on your hair strands. The overuse of these tools will eventually burn all your cuticle layers away, causing your hair to become subject to all kinds of hair disorders, resulting in severe and even chronic loss of hair.

Black women say, "White women can curl their hair every day so why can't we?" Well, ladies, you are missing a very important point. It is not that black women can't curl their hair every day, it's that we don't protect our hair when we do. Before the average white woman curls her hair, she will shampoo, condition, and even use a leave-in styling product on her hair. Now, is this because a white woman cares more about her hair than a black woman? No. Think about it—the average white woman has relatively straight hair and a pretty normal amount of active oil flowing from her scalp. They must shampoo before placing any heated styling tool on their hair because if they don't, their hair will become greasy.

On the other hand, the average black woman tends to have kinky dry hair and the scalp does not appear to have the same flow of oils. When she curls her hair every day, she feels it will give her a better style, and will apply oil to the hair before curling, never worrying about oily hair. Many black women feel that their hair looks better being curled each day. So, in most cases it is a matter of how a woman's hair looks and what keeps the style fresh. In any event, you must pay more attention to your hair care.

### Rules for using heated styling tools

Never blow-dry your hair from wet to dry. Instead, apply a leave-in conditioner to your hair strands, finger comb it through, then allow to air dry for five minutes before proceeding with the blow-dryer. By doing so you are allowing your cuticle layers to become more compact, thereby increasing the elasticity. Good elasticity is vital in preventing hair loss while blow-drying.

Never curl hair that has not been freshly shampooed and conditioned. Dirty hair will burn easily.

Always keep your curling iron and blow-dryer set on medium. Purchase an oven heat gauge so that you can keep a check on the temperature of your curling iron, pressing combs, and hot rollers. Never use a curling iron, a pressing comb, or hot rollers that are heated past 150°. Never leave your curling iron on for more then five minutes prior to using it, and always check to see if it has overheated. In other words, do not plug your curling iron in until you are ready to use it.

Avoid using more than one direct heat source for each style. For example, try allowing your hair to air dry overnight while sleeping on a satin pillowcase. Then curl your hair the next morning, eliminating the use of the blow-dryer. If you press your hair, avoid the curling iron all together. Use a moisturizer instead of an oil in order to prevent overheating of the hair cuticles, then apply Oil Sheen in a Jar to the ends and roll the strands. You can use sponge rollers; they come in all sizes, from very small to extremely large, and are even easy to sleep in. When using sponge rollers, it is very important to remember not to allow the hair and hairline to pull, and that you must wrap end papers on rollers prior to rolling your hair. Never allow the sponge to touch your hair, because the sponge will do just what a sponge is supposed to do, soak up moisture. It will also be too harsh on cuticle layers. All the things that I have mentioned can be applied to relaxed hair as well as natural.

When using heated rollers you must not be deceived into thinking that the rollers don't get as hot or somehow are less damaging than a curling iron. On the contrary, hot rollers can be more damaging because it is very hard to monitor or gauge how much heat the rollers produce. Think about it—when hot rollers are applied to your hair you allow them to cool down before you remove them. This uncontrolled heat sits on the strand and consistently burns into the cuticle layers, causing damage and resulting in strand thinning.

## Style alternatives

The use of any styling tools involving extreme direct heat—such as a curling iron, blow-dryer, hot rollers, or flat iron—should be avoided as much as possible. Following are some alternative style choices you may want to try. Remember that these are only a few suggestions; you can be creative and come up with your own. You may also want to consult a stylist that specializes in your hair type. Don't forget to use support products (moisturizer and oil).

Here are four suggestions. Use sculptor setting lotion in amounts determined by your style choice:

Apply five to twenty drops of setting lotion (depending on hair length) on natural hair, then twist or plait. Let air dry naturally if desired, you can let your hair dry overnight, sleeping on a smooth, satin pillow. Apply moisturizer, then press.

Apply three to ten drops of setting lotion (depending on hair length) on relaxed hair, then set or wrap hair.

Apply ten to thirty drops of setting lotion (depending on hair length) on natural hair, then create twist-braid styles and curly afros.

Apply twenty to fifty drops of setting lotion (depending on hair length) on relaxed hair, then style into French rolls or finger waves.

### Holding your style in place

Sculptor misting spray is an optional part of your style program. If you choose to use it, be sure that the product you choose has a low natural alcohol content. Never use spritz or any stiff holding spray. These products will cause a hardening of the cuticle layers, resulting in hair breakage.

## How to Dress the Hair and Scalp for Bed

You must prepare your hair for bed. Doing so will prevent your hair from drying out while keeping your hairstyle in place. It is not always necessary to cover your head or tie your hair up. This is only important if you have a close fitting hairstyle. Just remember only to allow your hair to be exposed to smooth fabric while you are sleeping, such as a satin pillowcase. This will prevent dryness and poor style retention. When traveling, take along your own satin pillowcase. Never use a sleep cap that has a tight elastic band.

Avoid rollers around your hairline, as they can cause too much pulling, which leads to breakage and hairline thinning. Instead, try pin curling. To pin curl, simply part a thin section of hair all around the perimeter of your head, then take a small piece of hair and roll it into a circle around your finger. Lay the circle of hair flat along your hairline, attaching with a small bobby pin, and repeat with the next lock of hair.

Never use cotton head wraps. Instead, use head wraps or scarves that have smooth fabric, and be careful not to tie them too tight.

If you have dry hair or night sweats, apply a small amount of moisturizer or oil throughout the hair. This will aid in maintaining moisture levels and prevent dryness.

## DRESS YOUR HAIR FOR THE OUTDOORS: WINTER, SPRING, SUMMER, FALL

Changes in the weather affect your hair just as they affect your skin. In the winter months or in dryer climates, you must always apply a moisturizer to your hair. Doing so will allow the hair to pull in whatever moisture is in the air and will keep your hair's moisture level balanced.

Spring will bring high winds that could tangle and damage your hair. Allowing your hair to blow in the wind can be safe if you prepare your hair. Remember your support product. Apply a moisturizer to your hair ends as well as the hair shafts. Then, after you come back in, be sure to carefully inspect your hair and use your fingers to remove all tangles. If your hair feels dry or brittle, lightly glaze the palms of your hands and apply more moisturizer.

The hot, humid months of summer are hard on a hairstyle, but not on your hair. Humidity will cause the moisture level in your hair to stay very high, which prevents dryness. This is one season where you will use very little moisturizer. But the heat will cause your scalp to sweat, and that will dry your hair and scalp out. Therefore, during the summer months you should shampoo and condition your hair more often, adding one per week if you are inactive, two if you are active, three if you are very active, and so on.

For your summer hairstyle, stick with styles that allow the hair cuticles to lay flat, thus preventing excess humidity from getting under the cuticle and causing the cuticle layers to puff and frizz. Setting the hair on smooth rollers will help. French roll styles are good choices. With natural hair, try more twist styles and avoid the use of any heated styling tools because your hair will turn back to a natural state as soon as you go outside. Then you will find yourself on a daily pressing cycle and you will burn your hair. To create a twist style, simply shampoo and condition as normal, then blot the hair with a towel to remove excess water. Apply a liberal amount of leave-in conditioner, then apply a liberal amount of oil to all your strands, finger comb your hair, and use the appropriate comb to comb your hair through. Make horizontal and vertical parts in your hair from forehead to nape and ear to ear in a crisscross pattern. Now take each small section and divide it into two and twist the hair until you reach your hair ends allowing a natural curl or flip to come in. Allow your hair to dry naturally.

During the fall months your hair will change a lot because the weather is so unpredictable. Be very hair and scalp conscious, listen to your hair and scalp, and see what it is asking for. I guarantee if our hair and scalp could talk, most of us would be deaf from the yelling and fussing that we would receive. The best rule to follow in the fall, as in all seasons, is to treat your hair and scalp with care, responding with the positive treatments that you are learning in this book.

# *Your Mind*

You cannot start the program and be successful until you have cleansed your mind.

*You must change your mind in order to have better hair. You are what you think and believe you are. You can achieve what you think and believe you can achieve.*

In order to have healthy hair you need to have healthy thoughts about your hair. You need to get to the root of the problem, and change the way you think about your hair and hair care in general. Start at the beginning—that is, wherever your problems began, you will find your new beginning.

In this section we will explore and expose the *mind* as it relates to our hair, *cleansing* any negative thoughts away and then *reconditioning* the mind with positive thoughts about our hair. We will look at many aspects of our life and expose how things, relationships, and situations affect the way we feel about our hair, which determines how we

**In order to have healthy hair you need to have healthy thoughts about your hair.**

treat our hair. You will see that this treatment of your hair will be reflected in how healthy your hair is, which will ultimately determine how your hair looks. You will come to know and understand yourself as a person, your hair type, and the many causes of hair and scalp problems. This will allow you to gain consciousness about your own hair, and at that very point, a level of awareness will arise within you. You will be able to freely individualize your needs (and not the world's needs) for your hair, giving your hair the care and attention that is necessary to truly fulfill the hopes, dreams, goals, and desires that you have for your hair. And then you will have better hair.

## UNDERSTANDING HOW YOUR MIND AFFECTS YOUR HAIR

You must first make the unconscious mind conscious, awakening to the fact that you have hair problems. Say out loud that this is not acceptable to you, and you will no longer be in denial or ignore your hair and scalp problems as if they if they will go away on their own. You will no longer pretend that you have it under control, saying things like "I cut my bad ends off so my hair can grow." You will not rely solely on a stylist, product, childhood lessons, or a dermatologist to solve your hair and scalp problems. You can and will gain the power to do something about it, using this book and all other sources that are available to you. You will take responsibility for what happens to your hair, which will determine how healthy your hair is now and for years to come. Your hair and scalp problems will only become worse if you do not do something *now!*

### I can control my hair!

You might get up each day and think about your hair problems, and become depressed and frustrated wondering why you are not able to solve them. You may say to yourself, I have tried this or that and nothing works. It is as if you have a handle on, or control of, many areas of your life, but each night when the day has ended you look in the mirror and cry wondering, "Why can't I control my hair?" Some of us are on a roller coaster ride because the hair seems to be healthy and growing and then the hair seems to stop growing and breaks off. You are not alone; this is a very serious and real issue that many black women are dealing with. Do not worry—by the end of the book you will say, "I can control my hair."

## Look inside

Over the years, many of my clients brought their complaints and questions to me, and after listening to thousands of women over a twenty-year period I realized something that they all had in common. None of the women wanted to look inside for the answers. Some blamed anything and everybody else for their hair and scalp problems. The women who took some of the blame never really looked inside to find the answer. The answer was there all the time, they just needed help to reach inside and find it.

## Negative thoughts

I define a negative thought or action as wrong, incorrect, out of order, or destructive. Negative and incorrect thoughts and habits that are imbedded within will not allow you to solve your hair and scalp problems, whether you have scalp problems, hair problems, or both. You must be conscious of the negative thoughts and habits that are causing your problems and preventing you from solving them. Many women go through a cycle of hair problems over and over again, because they cannot think past the negative thoughts and habits they have about their hair. You must get past that so you will be free to succeed.

Negative thoughts become habits. Poor hair care habits come from acquired negative thoughts and myths that become destructive

**I define a negative thought or action as wrong, incorrect, out of order, or destructive.**

and automatic. There is no room or pathway for the correct and positive, so your mind must be completely cleansed of every negative thought about your hair. Cleansing the mind of all incorrect and negative thoughts will clear a pathway and make available space in your mind and circle of thoughts for the correct and positive thoughts that are needed in order to have a successful hair and scalp care program.

## Poor Hair Care Is Second Nature

*We all are creatures of habit.* Habit is the function of our subconscious mind. You *learn* or become *educated* by consciously saying and then doing things over and over again until tracks are established in your subconscious mind. This is habit in action. For example, when you say, "I have bad nappy hair that won't hold a style, so I got my hair relaxed or pressed as straight as possible," your subconscious mind held on to that because you first said it then did it.

You felt correct and comfortable saying these things. You never knew that a simple and common statement could lead to serious hair problems. Think about it: the automatic, habitual action of your subconscious mind took over. First you told your mind that your hair is "bad" and nappy, and as black women we all know that is a negative thing to say about anybody's hair. Then you physically went out and relaxed or pressed your hair as straight as possible, resulting, whether you knew it or not, in some level of chemical damage or burned strands. I know that you did not look at it that way, because you surely never meant to cause any harm to your hair, but your lack of education on the dangers of the overuse of chemicals and heat on your strands caused the problems.

First, I will show you how to look inside and think more positively about your hair—for example, nappy, or as I like to call our hair "kinky," is not "bad hair." It has more body, bounce, fullness, and shine, and does not break. And, think about how much better the scalp feels when the hair is not relaxed or pressed as straight as possible. Second, had you educated yourself you would have

> **I will show you how to look inside and think more positively about your hair—for example, nappy, or as I like to call our hair "kinky," is not "bad hair."**

known that when 100 percent of the curl pattern is unnaturally relaxed from hair it becomes overprocessed. And, when you press your hair "bone slick" straight you are burning important top layers of your strands.

Wow! I know what you are thinking—how were you supposed to know all of that? I know, had you known better you would have never put into action such a negative thought that caused a negative act. But do you see how easily *poor hair care* becomes *second nature*, a mere reaction of your subconscious mind to your thinking? You

**You can only think into action what is already in your mind, so it is your responsibility to have the correct thoughts through education before you act.**

can only think into action what is already in your mind, so it is your responsibility to have the correct thoughts through education before you act. And, don't say that it was your stylist's responsibility to know. Remember, you are not to solely rely on anyone for the health of your hair. Don't worry, just exhale—by the end of this book you will be empowered to take the responsibility for the health of your hair.

*Why do we think that we can never have better hair?* There are many reasons why we think and then do negative things to our hair resulting in hair problems. We will expose many of them later in this cleansing of the mind in order to have better hair.

## Your Relationship with Your Hair

Having a good and positive relationship with your hair has many benefits, and is the key to having better hair. The way to do this is to make your hair problems personal. We know as black women that we have a history of political, cultural, and professional issues that have been and are still hanging over our head in relation to our hair. But in order to truly have better hair, we have to look at the personal—not the outside—destruction that we put ourselves through. This personal destruction is blocking and preventing us as a race from having better hair. So, let's make it personal—learn about you the person, then you can learn about this spiral thread-like substance, your hair.

Let's start by going back as far as you can remember to the first time that you became aware of hair and how important it was to you as a girl. Remember your first doll and how her hair would be when you first got her, all neat and in place. It was one of your first impressions of how hair should be. You probably got a small comb and brush to use on her hair to keep it neat and in place. Remember when you stopped playing with that doll and months later you found her

**Now try to remember the first time you noticed your own hair in the mirror. You looked, you touched it, then you smiled and thought "This is my hair, thank God for my beautiful hair." Or was it different?**

under the bed or in the bottom of the toy box? Her hair looked out of place and messy and strands began to fall out. So, you decided that you wouldn't worry about it because you would get a new doll next holiday. You said, since her hair is messed up (damaged), you would shave or cut it off and let her wear a short style. Even then, although you were too young to realize it, you placed a thought in your mind that if hair becomes damaged you can just cut it off and start over. You were too young to accept and take the blame for the damage, and admit that you were responsible, forgetting the fact that the only reason your doll's hair began to look like that was because you stopped taking care of it.

Now try to remember the first time you noticed your own hair in the mirror. You looked, you touched it, then you smiled and thought "This is my hair, thank God for my beautiful hair." Or was it different? When you looked in the mirror did you like your hair? Did you think it was pretty, or did you wonder why your hair was not like your sister's, friend's, or the little girls' on TV? Maybe someone told you that you had "bad hair" in a roundabout way. Maybe you had an aunt, sister, grandmother, or even your own mother, who told you that you had "bad hair." Even the times you thought that your hair was looking good, maybe after it was just combed, they seemed always there to remind you what they thought about your hair, saying things like "Girl, you know you got that bad stuff."

I remember that when I was growing up my mom always made us feel good about our hair. She would "water wave" our hair into a style, (you remember "water wave hair": first mama would take "grease," pile it on our hair, dip the brush into a jar of water then brush our hair and the waves would somehow just appear). Mama started "water waving" our hair at birth. Mama would never let us get our hair pressed until we reached a certain age. I remember begging to have my hair pressed to be like my older sisters, but my mama would say, "Don't rush, you have good hair and pressing will eventually mess up your hair."

My mama had seven girls and our hair always was neat and in place. She took the time to make sure of that. She said her mom always told her that she had "bad hair" and it made her feel bad about her hair. She told me she was so hurt that she prayed and told God if he blessed her with girls that she would never make them feel that they had "bad hair." I thank God for mama's prayers. I also thank Him for blessing my mama so that she could take that negative experience about her hair with her own mama and dispose of it so that she did not make any of us feel bad about our hair type.

I remember the first time my dad said something to the effect that one of my sisters had "bad hair." He asked my mother why my sister's hair was not like my other sisters' hair. My mama got so mad at him and said point blank, "It is because her hair is different from her sisters' hair, and there is nothing wrong with her hair." He never asked that question again. Although our hair varied, we all accepted our hair in a positive way. Even when "nappy hair" was mentioned, nobody felt that they really had "bad hair." And even today as adults when we have those Sunday family dinners at mama's house, we sometimes talk

**Thank God for the many moms that were blessed with understanding the importance of making their little girls feel good about their hair.**

and laugh about our "hair combing" days and the many things that mama taught us about our hair. Mama would tell us how she knew (as she put it) "what kind of hair each of her seven girls had." Mama not only never made us feel bad about our hair, she also would never allow anyone else to say anything negative about her girls' hair in her presence.

*Thank God, then forgive.* Thank God for the many moms that were blessed with understanding the importance of making their little girls feel good about their hair. If your mama, dad, aunt, or any other family friend or member consistently said negative things that made you feel bad about your hair, these things may have stuck with you and somehow lead you to believe that something was wrong with your hair. You must understand that, if someone said negative things to or around you about your hair, then those things were most likely said to them as a child and are being passed from generation to generation, so forgive them.

### Who is to blame?

As a people, we put far too much blame on the world outside for our hair problems. We think that people of other races are saying bad things about our hair, like "Black people have bad hair." I think it is time that we understood, believed, and came to know that we have

**As a people, we put far too much blame on the world outside for our hair problems.**

the power and have always had the power to determine what we feel about our hair. We should not allow other opinions to matter. Whether we want to admit it or not, the bad feeling about our hair came from within our own race, and in most cases from within our own families. Most black families were raised to have strong family beliefs, and once we believe something about or within our race, it is difficult and almost impossible to change our minds, negative or positive.

When it comes to our hair, there are many beliefs that we must change in order to have better hair. Oh, I believe that there are people that don't understand our hair, and some may say negative things about our hair out of ignorance, but they are the minority, studies and research have proven that. So, let's continue to look inside. Whether you had a "bad hair" experience from your mama, dad, other family members, or friends, it had some effect on you.

The way to know how it affected you is to focus on how you feel when you remember what was said to you, or what you heard about your hair or our hair type. Look at how much of what was said

**When it comes to our hair, there are many beliefs that we must change in order to have better hair.**

and what you heard stayed with you, how much of it you came to know and believe. Now ask yourself how much of what you remember hearing about your hair type was positive and how much was negative. Now answer this question: did you like your hair as a child, and do you like your hair as a adult?

## What happened?

I have been blessed to have helped many women through their hair problems. And I have found that women who hated their hair as a child not only had negative things said while growing up, but negative things were also done to their hair. Now, as you read keep in mind my definition of negative. *I define a negative thought or action as wrong, incorrect, out of order, or destructive.* Some grew up with a young mom who did not want to take the time with their hair, so they stayed in braids or gel pony tails. The child always heard things like "with mama's work load I don't have time to do your hair, so I need you to wear this style for a week or so." The style was usually one her daughter did not like, was too tight, or made her scalp itch and was not combed or shampooed for days or even weeks. Some stated that they grew to like the styles, thinking that if mama said it then this is how my hair is supposed to look. We must be careful with what we say to our little girls about their hair and how we treat their hair.

### Beauty shop drop-offs

Many moms would just drop their almost babies off at the beauty shop saying to the stylist, "Her hair is too much for me to handle, I can't do nothing with that bad hair," and just trust their stylist to take care of their little girl's hair. In a large number of cases, the child was passed over and just sat and waited forever for a turn to have her hair done. Some seemed to be put on display, with everybody coming up to touch their hair and give their opinion about what kind of hair that child had, "good or bad," as if the child was deaf. Little did they know or care that the child was taking it all in. And when the mom finally picked the child up, which was usually at the close of the day after she got all of her shopping done, she never knew why the child was sad. Many moms would ignore the child or not question the stylist, saying in front of the child, "She's OK, she is just being spoiled; she will be fine after I buy her a hamburger." All that mom was concerned about was how "cute" she thought the child's hair looked.

**We have a generation that does not know and has never seen their own hair in its natural state—think about it.**

I have interviewed many moms who were in tears and filled with guilt after their child had a bad beauty shop experience, but usually only in cases where hair loss occurred. I have treated children as young as thirteen months for hair loss and scalp problems after a mom trusted her baby to a stylist who relaxed her hair. Many stylists do take the time and patience needed to work with and care for a child's hair, but many will not. (By the way, thirteen months is too young. I will address the issue of how young is too young later.)

I would like to put this thought in your mind. We have a generation that does not know and has never seen their own hair in its natural state—think about it. I am not trying to lay a guilt trip on any mom, and I know that you did not know better, but now that you know, pass the word to other moms and do better. Moms must take the time to teach our little girls about their hair type—how to care for it, how beautiful it is, and how important it is to make others respect their hair. We never know how it will affect them later.

## Negative education leads to negative habits

Many women have bad habits, like shampooing only every two or three weeks; these habits came from how they were taught. You also have women who will wear a gel style for weeks, or braids for months until they almost rot off their head, saying, "I don't have time to fool with this nappy stuff," "Anyway, this is an easy, carefree style for me to take care of," or, "My hair grows faster with this style." Often, little or

**Many women have bad habits, like shampooing only every two or three weeks.**

no care or consideration is given to the hair or scalp while wearing these so-called "easy, carefree styles," (and, by the way, the hair does not grow faster). Many women will sit in a salon for hours waiting to have their hair done, rush home, call their girlfriend, and talk about the stylist and how unprofessional she was, only to go through the same thing again the very next week.

Now look back and try to make the connection. Can you understand that many bad hair and scalp care habits are passed from one generation to the next? The things that I have just talked about are things that echo some action from childhood. I will talk more later about the incorrect habits as well as myths that many black women grew up with and still believe to this day.

### Sneaky, subtle, seems almost harmless

Many women hate their hair as adults, and only seem to like their hair after it is changed from its original type. Many spent their teenage years, and now their adult life, going from one style to the next, never really satisfied. I found that among these women many would say things like "I hate my hair," or "I have always hated my hair." As they became adults, many would unknowingly do damaging things to change their hair, causing it to break, and then they would cover and hide their now-damaged hair with "added hair" such as braids, weaves, or even a wig (the most famous hair cover-up is braids). At the end of the day they still were not really satisfied

> **Many women hate their hair as adults, and only seem to like their hair after it is changed from its original type.**

and would become depressed and say, "My hair has stopped growing," or, "My hair only grows when I cover it."

Often, women never look back at the trail of destruction and never learn that their hair was made uniquely suited to fit them, and all they needed was to learn to embrace their hair type, learn how to take care of it, and give their hair the proper care and attention to be healthy. For many women, negative thoughts are embedded in their subconscious mind and need to be cleansed away and replaced with positive education.

### Sometimes hair problems come later in life

Women who like their hair usually liked their hair as a child and had positive people around them who had more positive things to say about their hair or about our hair in general. These women seem to have had no hair problems as a child, only later in life. My studies on this category of women lead me to believe that this is the largest group of women, they probably have the most hair problems, and they have stayed in denial the longest about their hair problems.

**Often, women never look back at the trail of destruction and never learn that their hair was made uniquely suited to fit them.**

These women believe everything and only what mama or their beautician said about their hair. Someone else had always taken care of their hair, told them when to shampoo and comb, and even what style was best for their hair. Many of these women were never allowed to shampoo or even comb their own hair.

Through the generations, black moms have been known not to let their daughters touch their hair. I remember my mom saying after she combed my hair, "You better not touch your hair and mess it up…" I have clients who didn't learn how to comb their own hair until they were sixteen years old. The life of their hair consists of: birth to age ten mama took care of their hair; age ten to age eighteen: beauty shop visits every two weeks with mama combing their hair on the off week. They never had to do or were never allowed to touch their hair as a child and teenager. Many of these women became dependent on someone else to take care of their hair, and make statements such as, "I can't do my own hair," or, "I don't do anything to my hair; I let my beautician do everything." These women now have daughters of their own and are making the same mistakes, but making them worse. Since these women never learned how to take care of their own hair, they don't know what to teach their daughters. This means that babies are being sent to the salon younger and younger.

**A change at some point had occurred with her hair and she and her stylist failed to recognize the changes.**

I have interviewed many young and older adults who were confused, wondering if they never had hair problems before, then why now. Some were confused about why all of a sudden they had hair problems after having the same beautician for years and getting the same hairstyle. Actually, the hair and scalp problems were brewing and just now came to light. A change at some point had occurred with their hair and she and her stylist failed to recognize the changes.

Something that was probably small progressed into a real problem. For example, your hair may not feel as soft as it used to, and you may not think much about it. But dry feeling hair is a sign of moisture loss within the hair strand, which left untreated will lead to more serious hair problems. I will talk more about moisture loss later.

Many women make statements like, "My hair was healthier when I was younger when mama or my old beautician took care of my hair." In their subconscious mind they believed that someone else could take better care of their hair. Many became what I call "salon dependent." As you got older you were forced to get involved with the care of your hair, but you did not know how. Mama is not there to "roll and oil" it every night, and say to you don't do this or that because it might hurt your hair. Mama was always watching over to make sure things were done just right. The problem was that although you can pick up on many things and learn positive things from mama and your old beautician, you were never really involved in the day-to-day care of your hair. This lack of involvement became negative later in life.

Now here you are trying to deal with your hair, you don't know your hair type, so you begin to experiment, but now you have changed and matured, and you want a new style. You may even try a new stylist that a coworker or college mate recommended. This person may specialize in style but not care, but you are thinking that she has a license and a large clientele, so she will be OK. Then, before you know it, the long beautiful hair that you always had begins to thin and break. So, you change, go to another stylist and she says, "Girl your hair has been damaged. You need to cut it off and start over." You never really looked at whether she was a hair care or a style person, again you were probably looking at the way she styled hair and at her large clientele. OK, so you let her cut your hair off, and one year later your hair is thinning and breaking again and on top of that you have developed an itchy, flaky scalp, and your relaxers burn. You ask what is going on and she says, "Girl you just have a sensitive scalp, and that thinning is coming from stress." At this point you either say no way, I let you cut my hair off, this is all new hair, and now it is your fault. Or, you believe her (because after all she is the professional) and continue to have hair and scalp problems until almost all of your hair is gone. Then she suggests that you let her weave some hair in until it grows back. Some stylists say things like, "After all, you are getting older and you will never have hair like you had when you were younger." Once again you change beauticians.

At this point, you become depressed and wonder what to do. You start thinking back to when mama and your beautician watched over your hair and how it was always healthy. So, you try to think what would your old beautician or mama do, or what did they use on your hair and scalp that made it so healthy. All you can remember is that big jar of "grease" that mama used when she combed your hair. The only reason you remember is because mama would let you hold the jar while combing your hair. You run out to buy it only to find that it is no longer made, or if you are lucky and find it, something seems to be wrong because it does not stop your hair and scalp problems. Your mama or old beautician is no longer around or you have in your mind that they are too old-fashioned to do your hair. In your mind you are thinking that you must find a new stylist.

You are now in a situation where your hair and scalp are damaged and you don't know what to do. A friend suggests that you go to a dermatologist, so you go, but are still having problems. At this point you don't know what to do, so you cut off your hair and go natural, saying, "If I can stay away from chemicals, I can grow my hair back and get rid of my scalp problems, too." And your scalp probably feels better to you without chemicals and your hair now covers your head and does not break as much. But you are still not happy, because you never learned how to embrace your own hair type in its natural state. You can't seem to manage your hair, so you run back to the chemicals and start all over again. You are so deep in denial and so unaware of how and at what point you got into this mess that you begin to just hate your hair.

### You need to stop the insanity and think

What has happened here is that you never learned about your hair and what your hair needed, so you did not know what to do. You went from mama to the beautician to the stylist. You were lost and could not find your way back home to healthy hair. The problem was you never knew the way in the first place.

### Thoughts don't just appear out of nowhere

There are many thoughts put in our minds by many sources relating to our hair type. Some seem to be part of our cultural beliefs and others are from what we see, hear, and read. You cannot go back and change your past hair experiences. What you can do is expose your past experiences and use them to find out why you feel and think a certain way about your hair. This will allow you to throw out the negative, thus clearing a pathway and making available space in your mind for the positive. This will change your automatic habit action within your subconscious mind freeing you to succeed in having healthy hair. You will be in control, you will hunger for the knowledge about how to get rid of scalp and hair problems, learning how you got in trouble in the first place and how you will never go back there again. You will then know that this is the hair type God blessed you with and God makes no mistakes. When someone tries to talk you into things that you now know will cause hair and scalp problems, you will simply say, "Sister to sister, been there, done that, got the T-shirt, I love my hair, and I ain't going back." As we now know, say, believe, and hold on to the incorrect things we are told about our hair, they will automatically be put into action, causing hair and scalp problems.

**You cannot go back and change your past hair experiences. What you can do is expose your past experiences and use them to find out why you feel and think a certain way about your hair.**

## TAKE THE RESPONSIBILITY

Your hair breakage happened because you let it happen, either because you did not know any better, or because you trusted someone else. In many cases you knew better, and wanted a particular style or "look" right then and there, not caring what happened. Sometimes we lie to ourselves and say, "Well, I guess this is what we have to do as black women in order to tame our hair or to make it look like something." Many will even say to themselves, "One time won't hurt," or, "I will just do this damaging thing this one last time."

Now, I know this sounds harsh, but let's look at how we are too trusting when it comes to our hair. How many times have you sat in a stylist's chair, or picked up a product off of the shelf, and not fully understood the side effects of the service that your stylist suggested or of using that product you just purchased.

**Your hair breakage happened because you let it happen, either because you did not know any better, or because you trusted someone else.**

Your stylist may have said something like this, "Let me bond this weave in your hair and your style will look better," or, "Let me retouch your hair every four weeks and your hair won't break." We all want to look our best so you said, "Sure, I trust you, go ahead and do it." You may have walked into your local beauty mart and picked up a bottle, box, or jar and it read "Super Grow, Long Hair in No Time." The girl on the box had long beautiful hair (and by the way it probably was not all her hair) so you said, "I want hair like her," and you bought it. You trusted it and thought it wouldn't hurt to try it.

Ask yourself, Did this really make sense to me? Did I understand the side effects of having the service that my stylist suggested, or using that product? What was said to you by your stylist or what you read on the box may have sounded good, but everything that

**Ask yourself, Did this really make sense to me? Did I understand the side effects of having the service that my stylist suggested, or using that product?**

sounds or looks good may not be good for you. You put your trust in your stylist, and that was not what you should have done, at least not in the way that you did. You should only trust when you have done your research on that stylist and know you can trust that she is qualified in every way to do that particular service, and you have researched that particular service or product and you know whether or not your hair can tolerate the application of such a service or product.

You may say it is the stylist and manufacturer's responsibility to provide the best in service and product. I agree that when you pay your hard-earned money you deserve and should expect the best, and you should be able to trust. We all know that does not always happen. It is ultimately your responsibility to trust only after you have explored every avenue that is available to you.

### Times you did the damage

What about the times when in your mind you knew that if you did a certain thing it would damage your hair or scalp and you did it anyway: you just let it happen. You knew that when you did it or had it done there was a possibility that your hair would eventually start to break or your scalp would dry out, but you did it anyway.

Now you are saying, "No way, I would never knowingly do harm to my hair and scalp." But many of us have in the past—think about the times you picked up a curling iron and curled dirty hair each and every day, and thought to yourself, "I know this is not good for my hair but I have to do it so my style will look good." How about that retouch that you got too soon because you were going out of town and you wanted a fresh look? Oh, and don't forget about that gel that we must have to lay our hair down; you used it knowing that it causes your hair to become dry and brittle, and your scalp to itch and flake like crazy. You did not care; at that point in time all you could think about was looking good for that moment.

At the end of the day it is still your responsibility to protect and care for your hair. One key to having better hair is not to overlook and be too trusting or to do things in a careless manner. If you want to stop your hair problems, you must start by taking responsibility. When you do that, you will be empowered and nothing can stop you from having not only better hair, but glorious hair.

## CLEANSING THE MIND

A major part of the cleansing process is to expose some of the myths buried in your subconscious mind. Many are things that we say on a daily basis. Some are things that we have heard for years. One of the goals of my studies on black women with chronic hair problems was to uncover statements, phrases, sayings, and myths that they had said or heard, believed, and came to know.

Here is a sample list of negative thoughts and myths that many black women believe.

1. I have bad hair.

2. My hair just won't grow.

3. My hair is so dirty, but it grows better when it is dirty.

4. My hairstyle only looks good when it is time to shampoo.

5. If I shampoo my hair that often my hair will fall out.

6. Braids and dreadlocks make my hair grow faster.

7. My hair breaks because of my nerve problem.

8. My hair will break because I need a retouch.

9. My hair breaks because I am stressed out.

10. My hair breaks because of the medication that I am taking.

11. My hair stopped growing years ago after a bad perm.

12. My grade of hair changed after I started pressing and curling.

13. Things are getting worse and will never change.

14. It is hopeless.

15. I don't know what to do.

16. Girl, I just have that kind of ("bad hair") hair.

17. We have to face it, we don't have hair like them.

18. Girl, you know your hair is just that nappy, "bad" stuff.

19. I don't know why God gave me this kind of hair.

20. They don't have hair problems.

21. Shampooing my hair too often will strip my hair.

22. If they go swimming, they don't have to do much to their hair.

23. I can't go running today because it is raining and my hair will turn back.

24. I can't work out because I don't have time to shampoo my hair.

25. I can't shampoo my hair; I am too busy.

26. I could not shampoo my hair because I was sick.

27. I could not shampoo my hair because I had out-of-town guests.

28. I could not shampoo my hair because my child, husband, mother, was sick.

29. I couldn't shampoo my hair because I was on my period.

30. I can't shampoo my hair because I just had a baby.

31. I can't shampoo my hair because my braids will get messed up.

32. I couldn't shampoo my hair because I got in too late.

33. I couldn't shampoo my hair because I was tired.

34. Grease will stop my scalp itch.

35. Grease will make my hair grow.

36. The only reason my scalp itches is because of stress.

37. If I grease my scalp my hair will grow.

38. She is the stylist; she should have known better.

39. I don't do anything to my hair; I just go to the salon and let my stylist take care of my hair.

40. It is her fault; she is the one with the license.

41. I know that she is young, but I put that perm in her hair because I could not comb her hair. It was just too nappy.

42. My hair is thick and nothing will hurt it.

43. My hair does not look good unless I curl it every day.

44. She has good hair so she will never have hair problems.

45. I know my hair can never look as good as hers.

46. My little girl has "bad" hair.

47. My hair will not lay down unless I use gel.

48. Gel grew my hair.

49. I gelled and braided my little girl's hair. It will last for two weeks or more, and it only itched a little.

50. It is too much work, and she has too much hair for me to do it every week.

51. I don't need to shampoo while I am wearing braids. All I need to do is use Sea Breeze, some mineral oil, and some braid spray.

52. All shampoos are the same so I will just use what everyone else is using or whatever is on sale.

53. I hate my hair.

54. I have always hated my hair.

55. Girl, I have growing dandruff.

And the list goes on—I am sure you have things that you can add.

### Can we talk?

You may be surprised at some of the things that I have listed, or you may not think that many of these things are negative. Many of you may say that if you happen to say some of the things that I have listed, you may be just kidding or saying them in a harmless way. Well, no matter what you think when you read my list, I can assure you that the things listed are negative. You should not think them, let them pass through your lips, or let someone else say them in your presence or in the presence of your child. Remember, a negative thought or action is wrong, incorrect, out of order, or destructive.

OK, you say that these things are not negative. I can easily prove to you that the fifty-five statements or phrases that I have just listed are negative. Let's talk about a few of them, starting with No.19: *I don't know why God gave me this kind of hair*. What if someone said to you or your child, "I don't know why God gave you that kind of hair." A statement like that would offend you.

How about No.25: *I can't shampoo my hair; I am too busy*. Making excuses about why you can't shampoo your hair will lead to more excuses, and then lead to your hair and scalp not having the care needed, which will eventually lead to hair and scalp problems.

Now let's look at No.39: *I don't do anything to my hair; I just go to the salon and let my stylist take care of my hair*. It is good to have a good relationship with your stylist and important to trust your stylist. I must again remind you that you must never rely solely on anyone to totally care for your hair. If you allow all of your hair care needs to be met by someone else you eventually will end up angry, surprised, and disappointed if hair or scalp problems occur.

We must look at No.51: *I don't need to shampoo while I am wearing braids. All I need to do is use Sea Breeze, some mineral oil, and some braid spray.* Your hair and scalp must be shampooed and conditioned on a regular basis. Nothing is going to clean your hair and scalp like shampoo, and even though your hair is under braids it must be conditioned properly.

And last, let's look at No.52: *All shampoos are the same so I will just use what everyone else is using or whatever is on sale.* All shampoos are not the same and you must keep that in mind when choosing one. You must choose one that works with your hair type. I will show you how to choose a shampoo later in this book.

Now, don't you agree that anything that offends you when said or has the potential to cause you harm should be classified as negative? Or, have you heard these things so often that your subconscious mind has held on to them and now you feel comfortable and correct hearing, saying, and even doing them? I have only exposed some of the most common negative things said, now you must participate. You must now make a list of negative thoughts, and things that you have thought or said about your hair. Only you can make this list, and it is very important that you do it because no one knows what you think and believe but you. By doing this you will expose your own very personal negative thoughts and feelings about your hair, and then you can permanently get rid of them once and for all. You will always know when these things are brought to you by some outside source, and you will not allow them to enter your mind because they are not correct. By exposing them and then ridding your subconscious mind of these thoughts you will make available space for the positive and correct. Believe me, you must now know how powerful the mind is, and how your thoughts can control your actions.

Remember, a negative thought or action is wrong, incorrect, out of order, or destructive.

Now, I want you to write your own very personal list of negative thoughts on a separate sheet of paper:

1. _____

2. _____

3. _____

4. _____

5. _____

Now burn it! _____

## RECONDITIONING YOUR MIND

Better hair is in your near future—just around the corner. We have just exposed many negative thoughts and actions that have been with you most of your life; now we will move on to the positive.

You can change your mind, and while reading this book, you *will* change your mind. As I said before, I will be right here with you. If you have the *desire* to stop your hair and scalp problems, you can *learn* and become *educated* on how to have better hair. Your desire is a part of the cleansing process, exposing, opening, and freeing your subconscious mind of all the negative thoughts and habits that prevent you from having better hair. This strong desire will cause you to focus and want to learn and become educated. You are already *halfway* there.

**If your mind is conditioned negatively, it can be reconditioned positively.**

If your mind is *conditioned negatively*, it can be *reconditioned positively*. Through raising your level of awareness and internalizing positive thoughts about your hair you will become *educated*, guaranteeing success in solving your hair problems.

## EDUCATION, NOT JUST INFORMATION

You may ask, how do you educate yourself in a way that will help you escape all your hair problems? There is a way, but you must first understand that there is a difference between education and information.

There is so much information. An abundance of hair product ads are targeted to black women. Top hair care professionals are holding summits and trade shows, claiming to have the answers to black hair problems. And, trade magazines have articles about hair problems in almost every monthly edition. All this available information, yet, we are still not *educated* about our hair and statistics show that hair problems among black women are at an all-time high. Just information is not enough.

## Hair products

You have hair products out there, but you don't know which ones to use, or which ones will give you better hair. No hair product will give you better hair if you don't believe that it is within your reach to have better hair. You most likely bought the product that had the best ad or price or gave you the trendiest style or best hold to your style. You should have bought the product that was best for the care of your hair and scalp. In some cases, you may have bought the right product, but you never used it properly or long enough to get the best results, or, after your hair got better, you went back to your old negative habits. You received product *information*, but what you needed was product *education*—education on what to buy, how to use it, how it is going to work to give you better hair, how long to use it before you can expect to see results, and how to prevent your problems from coming back.

## Hair care professionals

Stylists across the country say that they can solve the hair problems of black women through more salon visits and more personal consultations, as long as the client will just do what he or she says. That is only a part of the answer—remember, you cannot rely on anyone else to give you better hair. You have to educate yourself, take care of yourself, and, ultimately, take care of your hair and scalp. Also, if you do not like your hair, and don't think that better hair is within your reach, even if you do go to the salon on a regular basis, and even if your stylist is giving you the right information, you'll be sabotaging your success with your hair along the way, either by skipping salon visits or disregarding good advice, or in myriad other ways. Many women are receiving information and not education from their stylist. Whatever your stylist is saying and doing is either not correct for your hair or you are not grasping and becoming educated on what he or she is saying.

## Magazine information

Magazines have articles on hair almost every month, including information on the latest hairstyles, quick fixes, and how to look like the next model or star. Magazines inform us on what's new, but it is just information and that is not enough. Information comes at us in such quantities and at such a fast pace that we either don't hear it, or in self-defense we tune out what is said. This creates a

**The bottom line is, in order to change the way you think, information is not enough— you must become educated.**

problem because you may be missing valuable knowledge that can help you. In my opinion, it is time that manufacturers and others in the hair care industry start making the effort and taking the time to educate women about their hair and scalp—not just inform them about a new product. This would turn the industry on its head, but an educated person buying a hair product will be a more loyal customer who will in return not only buy that product over and over again, but will tell her friends to buy it as well. Then everybody wins.

The bottom line is, in order to change the way you think, information is not enough—you must become educated.

Information means something that is told to you. Education means learning—those things that you come to know, to hear, and to memorize or internalize. So, you can be *informed and told something*, but never *learn, memorize, or come to know it*.

Many of you have actually been *negatively educated* about your hair. You have learned and come to know the negative, become dependent, and gone into denial. It is now time to focus on the positive things about your hair. I will help you put positive thoughts in that now available space in your circle of thoughts.

## Positive affirmations

Let's start with a *positive affirmation*. I will give you complete step-by-step instructions on how to care for your hair and scalp; but, first things first. I want you to say to that person in the mirror each day something that will affirm and place you in a positive direction about your hair. It may seem silly at first, but it is very important that you do this until your subconscious mind comes to know that better hair is within your reach. Remember that to become educated is not to be told something (that's information), but education is something that you hear, memorize, and come to know.

Say a positive affirmation each day about your hair to yourself, preferably first thing in the morning and while looking in the mirror.

Thank God, believe, have faith, and each day say to yourself:

"I am not and will not be an obstacle in the way to solving my hair problems."

"I don't think and will never think of myself as powerless to overcome my hair problems."

"I am and will stay relaxed within my body, mind, and spirit, believing that my subconscious is open and is now becoming educated in solving my hair problems."

"I know that I have the power to face any adversities that come my way."

"I am empowered."

"Education and desire are establishing a new habit pattern in my subconscious mind."

"My habits and actions are now and will continue to be positive, correct, in order, and constructive."

"I am benefiting greatly and my hair is better."

You must now, at the same time, become educated. You must learn, memorize, and come to know that you have the freedom to choose a good habit or a bad habit.

**Education is the brush that will paint a picture of healthy hair in your mind.**

In fact, you are the only one who has full control of what you do and think. Choose to research your hair type, hair products, and what is good and what is bad for your hair and scalp. In doing so you are automatically choosing to understand your hair, and that understanding will allow you to learn to love your hair. Then you will only choose the products, styles, and care that are best for your hair.

Education is the brush that will paint a picture of healthy hair in your mind. You are now free, and you now have a hunger to learn. You now know that it is possible to have better hair. So, you will only hear things that are positive and correct about your hair. You will sift through information and only hear what is correct, and if it does not sound correct and does not make sense or not prove to be the truth, then you will not believe it.

Whatever mental picture, backed by faith in God, is held in your conscious mind, your subconscious mind will bring to pass. Visualize your hair and scalp in the best condition. Your scalp does not itch, flake, or feel tender or sore. Your hair does not break; it is not dry, brittle, or dull. You have hair that is at the length, fullness, and style that is best suited for you. You love your hair. You now have better hair because you are educated on how to care for your hair.

Use the following affirmations as well. Don't worry at first if you are not doing all the actions named in these affirmations right away. By the time you finish this book, you will have created positive and constructive habits and you will have better hair.

"I identify myself with my own aims and goals. Better hair is within my reach. I see it and now I identify with it. Everything that I do that relates to my hair is **"I have good hair."** positive and correct because I am reaching my goal of having better hair. I am there. This is me."

"I have good hair."

"God made my hair and God makes no mistakes. My hair is good; it is made to suit me. My hair strands are the correct shape and size to fit my hair follicles and my head. When I look in the mirror at my hair I think, 'What beautiful hair God blessed me with.' And when someone says something negative about my hair I will not hear them. I won't believe the negative statements, and I will not take on the negative things that they are trying to tell me. It is too bad that they can't see how healthy and beautiful my hair is."

"My hair will grow longer."

"My hair is becoming longer because I am now taking care to condition my ends and hair strands. I am no longer using overheated styling tools. I am no longer using damaging products that dry out my hair. Now my hair does not break and I can have longer hair."

"I will shampoo and condition my hair on an as-needed basis."

"When my hair and scalp are dirty I will shampoo. I will not wait for any stereotypical time set by others for shampooing my hair just because I am a black woman. I will shampoo my hair on an as-needed basis. I will adjust my shampooing regimen and shampoo more often depending on how active I am. I will shampoo my hair each time after a swim, and after I work out and sweat. My hair needs to be conditioned on a regular basis and I will do this. I will not say I cannot shampoo my hair because I am too busy or don't feel like it, or just to hold on to and save or keep a style. I will do correct things because I have learned and come to know that by doing so I am planting the correct seeds of health into my hair and scalp."

"I love my hair."

"I will today and each day choose to care for my hair and scalp. The choices that I make in caring for my hair and scalp will be correct and good. I will never wish that I had hair like someone else. I am free to stay natural or cut, color, relax, braid, or dread my hair— as long as it is my choice and I first educate myself on my choice."

"I can do it!"

"I am now empowered; my mind is changed. I am not afraid. I am doing it. I have better hair."

"I am empowered to prevent my hair problems and to succeed at my seven-week program, and I will succeed because I am educated to think first and then do things in a correct way."

"There is no need to be afraid. I will stay on my better hair care program for seven weeks and have success in getting rid of my hair problems. After I complete the seven-week program I will follow the maintenance and prevention program, and I will take care of my hair and scalp and prevent my hair problems from coming back. I have hair that is better now and I will keep my hair healthy now and for the years to come because the infinite power within has empowered me to do so."

## EMPOWERMENT VS. FEAR

You may find that the first thought that will come to you when you begin to recondition your mind is fear. When you doubt if you can stay on this seven-week program, or worry about the success of your hair care program, you are experiencing *fear*. When fear knocks at the door of your mind *stop*, now *think*. Always remember that the solution lies within the problem. Your hair problems are caused by the incorrect things in your mind—lack of education about your hair, negative thoughts, then acting on those incorrect things or thoughts, or allowing someone else to act and do incorrect things to your hair. In other words, the solution to your hair problem is always going to be simple—don't do incorrect things or allow incorrect things to be done to your hair and scalp, and you will have better hair. Period. End of discussion. This seven-week program will get you through the transition and set you up for better hair for life, not just better hair in the short-term.

**Always remember that the solution lies within the problem.**

### The up-and-down cycle

Sometimes between that roller coaster ride of damaged, then healthy, then damaged hair, you probably heard this small cry in your mind for you to do the right thing and care for your hair. You just ignored it and went ahead with something damaging. But don't worry, just exhale, and remember that your newly cleansed and reconditioned subconscious mind will not be a small cry, but a loud voice that will say, "I can and will do it." You will instantly become aware and you will do only the right thing. The only fear that you should have is that if you don't do the right thing your hair problems will start all over again, and that's a fear you must have. You are now feeding your mind with the correct and positive, and your mind will control your action—it's really that simple. You are now learning, so you do not need to be afraid. Fear does not have to be a part of your hair care program. Remember, part of your fear comes from the unknown and ignorance. Those things cause you to fail. After you read this book, you will no longer be ignorant about hair and scalp care, so you have no reason to be afraid.

## Pitfalls

Part of reconditioning your mind is to understand that there are things that will cause you to have a setback, if you let them. I call those things pitfalls. People who are around us each day can have an effect on us and our lives, and on the way we think, feel, and act. You have to decide how much you are affected by other people. Remember, you are the only thinker in your universe; you control the way you think, feel, and act. God has blessed you with the freedom to do that. Someone can tell you something, but it's up to you to hear them or believe what they say about you or your hair.

**You must be aware that just because you have this new attitude about your hair, the rest of the world may not feel the same way. Do not let this be a pit to fall into.**

When you are on your seven-week program you may for a period of time stop using a relaxer, and when your new growth starts growing in you should start to celebrate. A family member or coworker may say, "Girl you need a perm, forget about that program." A statement like that could ruin your whole day—if you let it.

This is a positive step for you and you are the one who will benefit from the steps that you take. You must be aware that just because you have this new attitude about your hair, the rest of the world may not feel the same way. *Do not let this be a pit to fall into.* The people who are close to you may be your greatest support, and sometimes they may not be. The only way for you to handle derogatory statements and actions from family, friends, and coworkers is simply to ignore them. If they cannot and do not agree with the steps you are taking toward healthy hair, that is their choice. It is your choice to continue with the program, knowing that the results you'll get will be worthwhile.

If this hair and scalp program is working for you (and it will), do not let someone convince you that it is not. In many cases you may not be able to talk about the new positive direction that you are taking as it relates to your hair. So, do not share your hair care program with anyone until you are comfortable with the idea that you may get a negative response.

You may wonder how someone could convince you that this program is not working when it is working. Remember that the people around us are people we see on a very regular basis. We trust them and in many cases we value their opinion. How many times have you said, "Oh, I can trust whatever he/she says," or, "I know if he/she says it to me I can believe it, because they are always going to tell me the truth whether I like what they say or not." Now, think about what you are saying. You are saying someone else knows you better than you know yourself. Personally, I don't believe that anyone knows me better than I know myself unless they are God almighty himself. In the past you may have come to believe that someone else can think for you, but your newly reconditioned mind knows better.

Just remember that you are the only thinker in your universe. You will only take into your mind the positive and constructive, not opinions from anyone who has not taken the time to look closely at all the steps that you are taking toward better hair. This person may be close to you in many ways, care about your well-being, and may have seen you go through hairstylists, products, and books, all the time watching you land in the same boat. They may have seen you fail in the past. Now they are convinced that you will fail again, and they may say things to you like, "I just don't want to see you get your hopes up." As I said earlier, they are thinking for you, but only because you let them. No one can think for you, and no one can act for you. Regardless of your past successes or your failures, don't give away your power now.

## Coworkers

For a moment I'd like to address a major pitfall my clients have encountered again and again. Many women have that one coworker who seems to be watching their every move and seems to have a negative opinion about everything they do. Each and every morning you get to work, you walk in the door, and there she is, just standing there as if she is waiting for you, with that fake smile. She starts with "Good morn——ing, how are you this morn——ing?" Your skin just seems to crawl. You are at the point of paranoia. Before you can get away from her here comes the daily hair question, "Girl, what is going on with your hair?"

Or, she may say or ask some of these things:

- So, you have a new style.
- I liked your hair better the other way.
- You must have a new stylist.
- Look who went to the beauty shop.
- I think that style makes you look older.
- Your face looks too round.
- Your face looks too thin.
- That style hides your face.
- Your wrinkles show up more with that style.

You just stand and you try to laugh it off as if something is funny when you know nothing is funny to you. You are feeling insulted. Why do you value her opinion so much? Deep inside you may not even like this person, so you may say that you would never value her opinion or believe anything that she says. This very person could be a pit to fall into. At this point you are saying to yourself, "No way this person could be in the way of my success in having better hair." I say, "Watch out."

Let's take a closer look. Each morning you know and expect this person to be there waiting for you. Each morning you give her your time even if it is only a few seconds, just enough time to insult you and possibly ruin the first part of your morning. Then you talk or think about it. You probably get upset with her, thinking, "She has a lot of nerve," or, "I am so sick of her opinions, and I wish she would just change and stop saying things like that." You may say, "Can't she understand that she is upsetting and offending me? How could a person be so mean?" She may not even be aware that she is offending you. Or, let's go as far as to say that there is someone who is that mean and is out to get you. Ask yourself what you can do about it. You have now allowed this person to enter your mind and control your thoughts about how you feel about your hair. You may be wondering what to do, and saying, "I come to work every day minding my own business, not bothering anyone, and there she is. How can I control this person, how can I stop her from saying such negative things?"

First, you need to know that you can't control her or what she says, and there is really no need to. You also should keep in mind that the only way anyone can have control of your thoughts and feelings is if you allow them to. As I said, you don't need to control or change her, even if you could. All you need to do is change your thoughts and make a firm decision on whether you are going to come to know the negative or the positive, and what you will accept and what you will not accept. You must decide what you will hear, and what you will not hear.

I know you are wondering how you're going to accomplish this. Simply put, the key word is to ignore her and not let what she says enter into your subconscious mind. Now, I am not going to make this hard for you to overcome, or make it bigger than what it is, and I am not going to let you do that either. You can and will do this without saying a word to her. The way to ignore is first to look at this coworker and say to yourself, "She is who she is and she will be that way until she decides to change." Now look at yourself in the mirror or in your mind's eye and say, "I am who I am and I have changed for the better. I know that I am a successful person and I am succeeding in my hair care program. This person has not taken the time to look at my hair program and doesn't really know me or what is important to me, so I will not place any value in their opinion of me and my hair. I have come to work today with confidence in myself and my efforts, and I will not try to control what comes from her mouth, but I will not let her control me. I will not be insulted or let her ruin my morning with something she said. I will not think or talk about what she says because I will not hear any negative words about my hair." Now, you must do this every day. Eventually she will get the message and just stop. People have a way of pressing things if they can get a response, and if they can't they will drop it. And if she does not stop she will be alone, because you are ignoring her.

## Negative statements

Be aware of negative comments that may be made directly to you or in your presence when starting this new positive hair care regimen. Some things that people will say to you are things that perhaps you even said and believed at one time. So, if someone says things that you know are negative, don't be hard on them, just remember that lack of knowledge is the cause. They don't know what they're doing. And always remember to pray for them because they don't know any better.

These are some negative statements you may hear when you start your hair care program:

- Black people should not shampoo their hair that much.
- Do you think that you are white?
- Girl, go get some weave because there is no kind of hair care program that can bring your hair back.
- Just cut your hair off and start over.
- You are spending too much time and money on your hair.
- If I were you I would never do what you are doing.
- Girl, you mean you are going to the beauty shop again?
- All that sounds good but I don't think that it will work.
- All hair products are the same, and none of them really work.
- This is just another way of making a lot of money off of black women.
- The only way you will ever have hair is if you go natural.
- Your hair will break if you don't perm it.
- That stuff that you are reading is only going to brainwash you and make you crazy.

This list goes on. Be ready and aware. The statements of others cannot hurt you except through your own thoughts and mental participation. Not everybody is going to agree with the steps you are taking. It would be a very kind thing on the part of the people in our lives if they would accept and believe as we do. But, their expectations are not necessary for the success of *your* hair care program.

## The Love/Hate Relationship that Women Have with Their Hair

How many times have you said, "I love my hair," and the next day, "I hate my hair." Some days your hair may style just the way you want it to and the next day it won't. You wonder why your hair won't hold a style.

Your hair may be reacting to the climate. For example, if your hair suddenly feels dry, the moisture level in your hair may have dropped, causing a dry, brittle feeling. This is very common when the hair is exposed to dryness in the air, usually in areas were the climate is dry or where there are cold winters. Your style will not hold if you allow it to dry out. Certain times of the year your hair may seem to grow and other times your hair may seem to break off. Your hair may be overexposed to the climate.

You may feel that your hair has a mind of its own. Don't hate your hair because it is not the same every day; learn to give your hair what it is asking for. As you are educated through this program, your elevated consciousness will help you to make adjustments in your approach to your hair, thereby giving you control over how your hair looks and feels, each and every day.

Learn to love your hair in its natural state before deciding to alter it. And, if you alter your hair in any way, be sure that this is what you want. If you make a mistake, don't hate your hair, or feel guilty. Make a choice to *educate* yourself so that you can take the correct steps and time to bring your hair back to where you want it to be. But, you must record this experience in your mind so that you do not repeat the same mistake again.

# Your Scalp

## UNDERSTANDING YOUR SCALP

Your hair grows from your scalp. The foundation to healthy hair is a healthy scalp, and education is the key to establishing and maintaining a healthy scalp. We must look at our scalp for what it is. Your scalp is skin. Your scalp is a part of the largest organ of your body, your skin. It has a need to be cleansed and cared for so that the pores of the scalp can be free to breathe, redevelop, and heal when needed.

### The epidermis layer

The scalp has two main layers of skin, and each layer has many sub layers. The top or outside layer is called the epidermis. This layer is thick and tough and protects the inner and more sensitive layers, called the dermis or true skin. When you look at your scalp you are looking at the outside or epidermis layers. The mouths of the hair follicles are housed in the epidermis. Take a look at your scalp, and notice that pinhole-like opening that your hair strand is growing from. That opening is the mouth of your hair follicle, and is the only part of the hair follicle that is exposed to the outside. You must never allow the mouth of the follicle to become filled with dust, dirt, debris, or other negative buildup. That is why shampooing when your scalp is dirty is a must. If you fail to do so, you eventually will have scalp problems that will lead to hair loss.

It is important for you to know that the epidermis layers have no blood vessels, therefore, these layers cannot bleed. Blood vessels are found in the inner dermis layers. When damage to your scalp causes it to bleed, that opens the door to more serious scalp problems. If you have ever had a retouch and your scalp got burned and bled, you may not have thought much about it because the skin most likely developed a scab and then seemed to heal. I remember when I started. I, like all the other stylists I worked with, saw chemical burns so frequently that we were nonchalant about them, just advising application of a little Neosporin. We certainly never intended to do long-term damage that could literally destroy a client's scalp.

**When damage to your scalp causes it to bleed, that opens the door to more serious scalp problems.**

### The dermis layer

The dermis layer houses the actual hair follicles. In addition to hair follicles found in the dermis layers, there are also sebaceous, or oil glands, sweat glands, and many delicate tissues and cells that are important to healthy hair growth. The oil glands in the dermis layer consist of little ducts that point toward the mouths of the hair follicles.

One of the invisible substances continuously secreted through the oil glands to the epidermis layers, to the mouth of the hair follicles, and on to the scalp, is called sebum. Sebum is important in keeping the scalp soft and supple. The scalp also secretes an acid mantle that is a mixture of a substance from the oil and the sweat glands. This substance gives the scalp its pH of 4.5 to 5.5, which is the normal pH of a healthy scalp. A healthy scalp is slightly acidic because of the acid mantle, and is lubricated by the sebum.

### You could be damaging your scalp and not be aware of it

The scalp is skin and skin is an organ that can be damaged. Take a moment and think about your scalp as you would the skin on your body. The skin on your body must be cleansed and cared for on a regular basis, and when doing so you exercise precautions to avoid products that will cause dryness and irritation to the skin. For example, if you cut, burned, or caused injury to your arm, you would care for and nurture the skin on

**The scalp is skin and skin is an organ that can be damaged.**

your arm back to a healthy state. You would take special care to keep the injured area clean. You would notice that as it healed it went through two main phases. First, your body's natural antibodies and any oral or topical antibiotics you apply would bring any infection to the surface. Secondly, after the infection is brought to the surface, the affected skin becomes dry and tight and itches like crazy. Even though it would itch immensely, you would abstain from scratching for fear of breaking the skin and reinfecting it.

*Well, the same healing process holds true for your scalp*. When the scalp (which, remember, is skin) is damaged from chemical burns, or burns from a pressing comb, curling iron, hot rollers, or any other heated styling tool, it must heal the same way your arm would heal. Your scalp can also become damaged from drying shampoos, gels, and other drying styling products.

Poor scalp care will, over a period of time, cause the outside layer of the skin to become bruised, thin, and eventually worn, exposing the dermis layers. At that time the scalp becomes sensitive and immediately tries to heal itself. Like the skin on your arm, the scalp first attempts to bring the infection to the surface. But in many cases the scalp is dirty and does not have the right environment for healing.

> **Poor scalp care will, over a period of time, cause the outside layer of the skin to become bruised, thin, and eventually worn, exposing the dermis layers. At that time the scalp becomes sensitive.**

Buildup of hair products, dust, dirt, and debris will house bacteria that will slow down or even stop the healing process. Unlike the skin on your arm, the skin on your scalp has not been given the opportunity to heal. So, the scalp becomes infected, and as the infection or inflammation tries to surface, it will often be accompanied by dryness, flakiness, and itchiness.

The natural reaction to this dry, itchy, flaky scalp problem is to scratch with fingernails or other sharp objects. This only prolongs the healing process even further and often causes more damage to the skin as the infection spreads. Keep in mind, too, that your fingernails are holding a countless number of germs, and when you scratch your scalp you are causing more problems. An area that was once a small damaged spot on the scalp may now spread over a large portion of your scalp, or even the entire scalp. Conversely, if you had taken good care of your scalp, a quick healing process would have been possible.

Nowadays many people label a damaged scalp as a "sensitive" scalp. At this point your scalp has become sensitive because of the wearing through of the epidermis layers. The cycle of damage will continue until you take better care of your scalp. Now, let your newly educated subconscious mind be your guide to a healthy scalp.

### Lifting the dandruff

For years, scratching the scalp, or as we called it, "lifting the dandruff," was a common part of the treatment of flaky scalp. I remember growing up and seeing many of my family members have their scalp scratched on a weekly basis. It was one of the many ancestral rituals that we held near and dear

**Never scratch your head with fingernails or other sharp objects.**

to our hearts. Often, immediate gratification and relaxation would be experienced from the constant sawing of the comb on their scalp. But a few days later, the scalp would began to feel dry and itchy again. Why? Part of the reason is that the scalp was trying to heal itself! People mistakenly believed that the reoccurrence of the itchiness and flakes was due to new dandruff; but, it was the epidermis layers trying to heal, and the more that the scalp was scratched, the more the scalp would flake and itch. The constant scratching caused further injury and opened the scalp to reinfection, eventually leading to one of the real unknown dangers, subsequent baldness.

Even later when I made the decision to become a stylist, I realized that many salons practiced this "scalp torture" not knowing the dangers. I was told by an older and more experienced stylist, and I must quote her exact words, "Baby, you just need to scratch that head real good and work that dandruff up, then you can shampoo it out and get rid of it." Afterwards, she instructed me to pour Sea Breeze on my client's scalp. The client would look as if she was in pain but would not say a word because she knew this was a standard treatment and just one of the many necessary evils to treat the scalp. I felt uneasy because I knew the client was experiencing discomfort. Sometimes her scalp would bleed a little. When I would ask if I was hurting her she would say, "It hurts and feels good at the same time." Occasionally clients would say, "I don't want my dandruff lifted today—my scalp is too tight and sore from the last time, but I will be ready in two weeks."

**I am now convinced that "lifting the dandruff" eventually caused high levels of scalp damage.**

I am now convinced that "lifting the dandruff" eventually caused high levels of scalp damage. At the time, we simply did not realize the damage we were causing to the client's scalp, nor did we pay attention to the fact that the more we scratched each week, the more the scalp would flake.

## Low-Level and High-Level Scalp Damage

There are two levels of damage that can occur to the scalp: *low level* and *high level*. The causes for these types of damages are innumerable. However, there is one thing that you can be sure of: if you damage your scalp, no matter at what level, left untreated *you will continue to have problems*. Many women will do negative things to their scalp and cause scalp damage as I mentioned earlier, but in many cases they don't understand why. Some are confused about why this is happening to their scalp or why this only happens at certain times of the year. You know, sometimes your scalp may seem to be dried out, then at the same time it will flake and itch for no apparent reason. You may say, "I put oil on my scalp but it is still dry." There is a reason why. Your scalp may be experiencing low levels of damage.

### Low-level scalp damage

With low-level scalp damage, you may experience one or more symptoms, such as a dry, tight, flaky, or itchy scalp. Low-level scalp damage can derive from many sources, and most of the time you never notice how your small day-to-day activities contribute to this type of damage. Two of the causes of low-level scalp damage are exposure to dry climates and sudden temperature changes.

Different parts of the world experience different climates. In some parts of the world, the winters are cold and dry, and in some parts winters or summers may be hot but still dry, and yet in other parts there may be considerable heat and humidity. Whether you have cold or hot climates, the skin will react negatively to dryness in the air. Have you ever noticed the difference in the appearance of your skin in dry climates versus more humid areas? In places where you have cold, dry winter months, the skin on the arms, legs, and other parts of the body typically will appear dry and "ashy," so women consistently apply moisturizing lotions to keep the skin soft and lubricated and to prevent cracking or chafing. On some cold, windy days, you may notice that your face will burn, then become rough and dry. Remember, the scalp is skin and your scalp can become very dry when it is overexposed to cold, dry weather. In many cases this can cause scalp damage. In these conditions, just as with the skin on your body, your scalp will become tight and dry, then it may flake and itch. Scratching the scalp only causes more damage. This dryness is a form of low-level damage and should not be ignored or aggravated by scratching.

Areas where cold, dry winters occur are further complicated by extreme sudden changes in the temperature. For example, in areas where you have cold, dry winters, your scalp often goes through a variety of extreme sudden temperature changes over the course of a given day. How? During a typical winter's night, many, after retiring for the evening, tend to keep their houses very toasty and warm, creating hot dry air. The next morning on your way to work, you probably go outside to warm up the car. Now you have exposed your scalp to cold dry air. Next, you go back into the house to finish dressing or wait for the car to warm up—hot dry air. (Are you beginning to see the big picture yet?) As you drive to work you're in what?—hot dry air. You get out of the car and go into the building, once again exposing yourself to the cold dry air. Now it's time to go inside to your warm building. After entering, you immediately lotion your hands and scratch your scalp. (Please note that when entering the warm building from the outside you properly add moisture to your hands to eliminate the dryness, while on the other hand, you scratch your scalp to ease the dry, itching feeling you are experiencing.) I have not yet even mentioned lunch breaks and stops that you make going to and coming from work. The multiple temperature changes that you have taken your skin through, which includes your scalp, creates dryness as the body works hard to stabilize itself with the environment. Changes such as these are primary factors in causing low-level scalp damage.

Even though you can't realistically avoid these changes in temperature, there are some remedies to alleviate scalp dryness. Just remember to shampoo on a regular basis, at least every three days. Now you may be concerned that shampooing more often will dry your scalp even further, but that will depend on your shampoo. Remember, your newly subconscious mind is open and now has available space for the positive. Let this information become education.

Use a shampoo that is acid balanced 4.5 to 5.5, which is the pH of your scalp. It is imperative to stick to a shampoo that is the same pH as your scalp—4.5 to 5.5—because alkaline shampoos not only fail to heal, but often add to or worsen the problem. What is an alkaline shampoo? Alkaline shampoos have a pH of 7 or higher and are detrimental to a healthy scalp. Be sure to look on the back of your favorite shampoo to determine the pH level. If not listed, contact the manufacturer immediately. Also, please be sure that your styling products, such as hair sprays, gels, and mousse, do not have a high alcohol content, which also can cause dryness and low-level scalp damage.

If dryness persists after using the proper shampoo, simply apply a pure oil (not grease) to the dry spots. These very simple treatments can completely eliminate low-level damage that occurs during cold dry winters. In this book's seven-week program, you will learn how to care for your scalp and prevent other low-level scalp damage. I will talk more about choosing the correct shampoos and oils later.

### High-level scalp damage

With high-level damage, the scalp becomes thinner and susceptible to more serious problems, including scalp infection. Instead of treating the scalp in a positive way during the low-level damage period, many women will, as I mentioned earlier, do negative things to the scalp, such as scratching. Many black women will treat a dry, itchy, flaky scalp by piling on "greases," such as Sulfur-8 or Glovers Mane, which seem at first to help some of the dryness, but then make the problem worse. Many of these products tend to clog and damage the surface of the scalp from which the hair extends, and subsequently house bacteria that can and will lead to scalp fungus. Although oil will assist in healing, grease products do not.

As low-level scalp damage evolves to a higher level, the scalp will become sensitive. Many will say, "I have a sensitive scalp," not realizing that the scalp is only sensitive because it has been damaged and has not had an opportunity to heal. At this time, almost any and everything the scalp comes in contact with that is not the same pH as the scalp itself will aggravate the existing problem. Then, when it is time for a chemical application such as a relaxer or color treatment, the now-sensitive scalp becomes more damaged and bruised by chemical burns.

## CHEMICAL BURNS

Chemical relaxer burns are high-level scalp damage. Chemical burns happen when the scalp has become worn and thin, usually due to improper scalp care. In many cases, the scalp has been exposed to high pH shampoos, improper application of chemical treatments, as well as overexposure to many chemical treatments. In studies that I conducted on the effects that chemicals have on the scalp and hair strands when improperly applied and left on for excessive lengths of time, I found that a chemical relaxer will completely dissolve scalp and hair strands. The scalp becomes thin, and oozing and bleeding may occur. At that point a visit to a dermatologist may be needed. Instead of treating the scalp and nurturing the scalp back to health, many women at this stage don't know what to do, so they turn to "sensitive scalp" or "no lye" relaxers. These chemicals only cover up the problem. I call them "the silent killers." Although you may not experience burning while "no lye" chemicals are applied to your hair, in most cases in the days following you will experience tightness, dryness, flaking, itching, and maybe even tenderness of the scalp. If left untreated, this type of scalp damage can cause serious scalp infections leading to high-level scalp damage and even thinning or baldness.

For years, many women have these "no lye" chemicals applied, not knowing that it may be adding to the problem. When they turn to their stylists for help, they realize that their hair care professionals also believe that "no lye" relaxers are milder than other chemicals. But all chemicals have

**For years, many women have these "no lye" chemicals applied, not knowing that it may be adding to the problem.**

the potential to cause harm, because they are chemicals. If a chemical is used properly by a trained professional, then your hair and scalp will not become damaged. When your scalp is healthy it should feel cool when you are having your hair relaxed. Although the relaxer is applied to your hair, at some point your scalp will come in contact with the relaxer. When your protective (epidermis) layers are intact and healthy, they will allow your scalp to resist burns during any chemical process. When poor scalp care is practiced and chemicals are rinsed improperly, the epidermis layers will not be there to resist chemical burns.

## DANDRUFF OR DRY SCALP

Although dandruff or dry scalp is very common, these small white scales are usually taken too lightly and considered a mild scalp disorder. Dandruff and dry scalp are very serious and could lead to high-level scalp damage. Left untreated they are guaranteed, although maybe much later in life, to lead to "surface baldness."

The nature of dandruff is not clearly defined by medical authorities, but dandruff is said to be an excessive peeling of the scalp. The surface cells accumulate on the scalp, instead of shedding and falling away, by literally packing inside and around the mouth of the follicle. These flakes or dead-skin scales can create a blockage within the scalp pores and a breeding ground for bacteria and even fungus that can cause a scalp infection.

After conducting a study on the scalp of black women and men, I found that in many cases people were using high pH shampoos, causing the scalp to peel. I also found in my studies that when high-pH shampoos were used, the scalp was worn down and the individuals complained of sensitivity and always suffered burns when chemicals were applied. Looking further into the scalp care regimen of those

**Dandruff and dry scalp are very serious and could lead to high-level scalp damage. Left untreated they are guaranteed, although maybe much later in life, to lead to "surface baldness."**

in my study, I found that many only shampooed every two, three, or even four weeks. Many of the participants also were exposed to dry climates and sudden climate changes. All of these factors are vital in keeping the scalp free from excessive peeling. The scalp will respond negatively and produce dry scales as a reaction to the environment and the healing process of the skin. The scalp was just doing the natural thing and trying to heal itself. Many who participated in my study found that their condition could be corrected simply by following the steps in my scalp program.

Before becoming involved in my study, many had made visits to several dermatologists and were told of various causes for their dandruff problems. The dermatologists would prescribe shampoos and creams to alleviate the problem. Also, the patient was told to shampoo daily. Many blacks would use these medicated products a few times and then stop using them, complaining that, although their scalp got somewhat better, their hair became hard and dry and broke off. When you tell a black person with dry scalp and dry, kinky hair to shampoo daily, you had better also tell them what to do with their hair, and how to care for it and prevent dryness. Many of the patients stopped using the prescribed products because they were afraid that, in addition to their scalp problems, they now had hair problems and thought that they were facing the possibility of losing all of their hair. When they stopped using the prescribed products, they found that their scalp problem persisted. The clients were basically caught between a rock and a hard place. If they used and followed what the doctor had prescribed, their hair was hard and brittle, but when they stopped, the scalp problem once again became an issue. Needless to say, my clients were frustrated and confused.

In my seven-week program, I give you simple, easy treatments to follow that have been tried, tested, and proven to work and that will help to create an environment for healing. These natural, safe steps will enable you to follow your doctor's advice as well as save your hair.

## One Woman's Story

A true story. I have treated many scalp problems and worked with many that were misdiagnosed—too many women find themselves in this situation. But there was one client who comes to mind whose experience I will never forget. This particular client, whose name is Ms. Avery, had one of the worse cases of flakes and itchy scalp that I had ever seen. Her scalp was almost completely covered with thick, white layers of flakes; the mouths of the hair follicles were being smothered. In addition to the scalp problem, her hair was falling out in handfuls. She was at her wits' end, desperate to find out what was going on with her scalp and why she was losing her hair.

The woman was willing to try almost anything. She had been to three different dermatologists, not to mention many stylists. Some stylists had tried and failed to come up with a treatment that would get rid of her problem, while others told her to see a dermatologist. Out of the three dermatologists she saw, one told her she had a fungus and gave her the appropriate medicated products for scalp fungus. But this product did not provide the woman with any relief. The next one told her that her scalp problems were due to poor diet and improper circulation, and he prescribed medicated shampoo, ointments, vitamins, and a special diet. But after three months of following the doctor's advice her scalp problems were still present and she was still losing hair. The last dermatologist was female and my client thought she might have found someone who would understand not only from a doctor's point of view, but also from a female perspective.

This doctor gave her a prescription and instructed her to apply and pack her scalp at night with a pasty cream medication. She was to sleep with this on her scalp overnight and in the morning (at least eight hours later) rinse, then use the prescribed shampoo. My client reported that she was afraid of the process and how dry her hair became, but continued to use it until she completed the entire prescription. She reported that this last doctor tried several other medical treatments to solve her scalp problems, but none worked. The doctor finally told her that she had tried everything that was medically possible. She told her she honestly could not help.

By the time the poor woman came into my center, after hearing about me through a friend, she was in a devastated state. After I looked at her scalp through the magnifying lamp and under a hand-held microscope, it was clear to me that she had scalp problems that involved more than dandruff or dry scalp. Luckily, I had completed a study on scalp flakes and how to treat the problem, and I had developed an effective treatment program that takes a more natural approach. Under the treatment program that I recommended to her, Ms. Avery's scalp problems are under control and she is no longer losing hair. With the right focus and the correct treatment, many scalp problems that seem impossible to solve can be solved.

Ms. Avery is one of a growing number of women who are suffering with scalp problems unnecessarily. Many go all their life with these types of scalp problems, and some lose their hair even to the extreme of baldness. There are only a few of us out there who have found treatments that actually work. I have been in this industry for over twenty years, and I have spent countless hours in research and study of both the scalp and hair, particularly on blacks. In order to help individuals like Ms. Avery, I believe that the cosmetology industry must do its part and change, adding the appropriate updated education on scalp treatments. There are numerous specialty licenses for professionals who want to specialize in scalp care and treatments. Manufacturers of scalp care products must also make an investment and a concerted effort to join the cosmetology industry in solving many problems of the scalp. If we do our part as professionals, I believe we will start to see fewer clients becoming patients.

I am not trying to say that the things that were prescribed to this patient were not medically sound. We need dermatologists to continue to do their job because they do benefit many. However, in fairness to many cases, and particularly in this client's case, it was time to look at the situation in a different light. We must begin to understand that not all scalp problems require medical attention. Many people, particularly African-Americans, go on for years with chronic and extreme scalp flakes and never get the help that is needed. I found that this is because either the individual did not try to get help, saying that "dandruff just runs in my family," or their dermatologist may have misdiagnosed the problem.

## Negative Buildup

Just because you see flakes on your scalp does not mean that you have dandruff or dry scalp. Many clients have come into my research and treatment center claiming to have dandruff. And I must admit, even to the most trained naked eye those flakes could be mistaken as dandruff or dry scalp. But, in many cases where an individual was told that they have chronic dandruff problems it turned out to be a misdiagnosis.

The scalp is the foundation from which your hair grows, and sometimes dust, dirt, debris, dead skin cells, and hair products become trapped in the scalp, causing a buildup. If the hair and scalp are not shampooed properly on an as-needed basis, and/or the hair products that you use are not water-soluble, then your hair and scalp will develop what I refer to as "negative buildup." Negative buildup develops on the hair and scalp and either will not rinse clean or will not shampoo out easily. Some conditioning shampoos are culprits in causing a negative buildup. Many black women will buy a so-called "conditioning shampoo" because it will make their hair feel soft and silky, not knowing that these "all in one" shampoos are not getting the hair and scalp clean. In a study, I found that some women who used "all in one" or conditioning shampoos complained of a flaky scalp and thought that they had dandruff. So, in addition to using the "all-in one" shampoo they would use a dandruff shampoo. This combination of shampoos left their hair dry and filmy, and left their scalp tight, dry, and even flakier than before.

Negative buildup looks like dandruff to the naked eye, but when examined under a microscope, it is not dandruff, but a substance that resembles minute pieces of trash. In some cases where an individual has piled on grease products to combat itchy scalp problems, the negative buildup resembles slime. This type of buildup will crowd around the scalp pores and create blockage at the mouth of the hair follicle. This blockage will cause scalp infection or high levels of scalp damage.

Scalp damage, no matter what level, should always be taken seriously. Low level damage will eventually lead to high level scalp damage and will cause problems with hair growth. Remember, your scalp should always look and feel healthy. Never ignore a scalp itch or a dry scalp because it could be the beginning of more seri-

**Just because you see flakes on your scalp does not mean that you have dandruff or dry scalp.**

ous problems. Always do a scalp inspection and listen to what your scalp is telling you by the way it looks and feels each day. By doing this, you will preserve your scalp and prevent disorders that may need medical attention.

## SCALP DISORDERS THAT MAY REQUIRE MEDICAL ATTENTION

Although low level scalp damage can be treated at home, high level damage must be treated in a salon and in severe cases may require medical attention. Some common scalp disorders that will require medical attention are ringworm, scabies, head lice, and scalp boils. Although these scalp disorders require medical attention, you must have a good hair and scalp care program to offset the side effects caused by using medicated shampoos and prescribed treatments.

Remember, your hair and scalp are connected, and anything that is used on the scalp must be closely monitored to be sure that it does not dry out the hair and scalp. In other words, do not solve one problem and create another problem. This is an important warning because many dermatologists have told patients who complain about hair problems after using scalp medication not to worry about their hair until the scalp heals. This statement has caused many clients to refuse the prescribed scalp treatments because they are not willing to sacrifice the style of their hair. As a result, their scalp problems got progressively worse.

**Remember, your scalp should always look and feel healthy.**

What should you do? You should first go to a salon that specializes in scalp care, and then let that scalp care professional tell you whether you need to see a dermatologist. Be sure to ask for recommendations. This will assure that you get someone who is sensitive to your needs. You are becoming educated on your scalp and how products may affect you. By the end of this book, you will be empowered to make the proper choices. You will know the value that research plays in finding out all the side effects of medicated scalp products. You will be able to be involved in how your scalp is being treated. You will find that education is the key that will open the door and allow you to enter into making the positive and correct choices. Then you will learn and come to know what to use to stop your scalp problems without having to sacrifice the health of your hair.

## CARING FOR YOUR SCALP

A healthy scalp starts with a clean and conditioned scalp. The basic requisite for a healthy scalp is cleanliness. A clean scalp resists a variety of scalp disorders. A clean scalp is also free from negative buildup. As you have learned, your scalp has pores and hair follicles that can become clogged and damaged, and since the hair grows from the scalp, proper scalp care is vital in encouraging consistent hair growth and in obtaining and maintaining healthy hair.

## GUARANTEE A HEALTHY SCALP AND PREPARE THE SCALP FOR HAIR GROWTH

Following are the steps that will give you a healthy scalp and prepare your scalp for hair growth.

### Shampoo on an as-needed basis in order to have a healthy scalp

Start paying attention to your scalp. Give your scalp what it is asking for. Just like the skin on other parts of your body, your scalp needs to be cleaned regularly. The skin on your entire body naturally sheds and replaces the upper part of its outside layer. The scales fall freely from your body in the shower and bath, onto your clothing, and will even dissipate in the air. Unlike the skin on the rest of your body, your scalp may not always have that same opportunity, particularly with women and men with hair longer than half an inch. And in cases where the hair is kinky, it is difficult for the cells to freely fall away no matter what the hair length. Your hair acts as a trap and causes the skin scales and other debris to accumulate. After three to four days, even a healthy scalp has a buildup.

Many people wonder how often to shampoo. The answer is: shampoo on an as-needed basis, when your hair and scalp are dirty.

**A healthy scalp starts with a clean and conditioned scalp.**

You should shampoo at least two times a week. Increase the number of times per week that you shampoo according to how active you are. If you are on a special scalp care program, you may need to shampoo even more. Don't forget to do your research.

### Never use sharp objects that will scratch your scalp

This includes combs, shampoo, brushes, ink pens, and any other things you are using to poke and dig at your scalp. Remember, scalp is skin and can be damaged.

### Protect the scalp from direct and extended exposure to the sun

Overexposure to the sun could cause sunburns on the scalp surface. In cases where the scalp has suffered extreme scalp burns, your scalp could develop scar tissue. Depending on the thickness of the scar tissue, it could create a blockage on the mouth of the hair follicle. This blockage will prevent the hair from growing through and baldness will occur. In many cases, your hair will not be able to protect your scalp from the sun's rays. You should always cover your head when you are going to be in direct sun.

**Do not overexpose your scalp to chemicals.**

Never chemically treat your hair when your scalp is damaged. Chemical burns are similar to sunburns and can cause problems that may prevent proper hair growth. Chemical burns will eventually lead to high level scalp damage. Always pay close attention and treat the scalp, bringing it back to health before chemicals are applied.

**Many people wonder how often to shampoo. The answer is: shampoo on an as-needed basis, when your hair and scalp are dirty.**

## THINGS YOU MAY DO THAT DAMAGE YOUR SCALP

Many negative things are done to the scalp that could discourage hair growth and cause scalp damage. When you do negative things to the scalp, your scalp has to recover or heal. You want to be careful to nurture your scalp. Following is a sample list of things you may be doing that can cause scalp damage:

- Not shampooing on a regular and as-needed basis
- "Lifting the dandruff"
- Shampooing with pointed tooth shampoo brushes
- Working out and not shampooing
- Piling so-called "hair growth products" into the scalp
- Bonding hair to the scalp
- Pulling bonded weave hair from the scalp

- Sewing and pulling weaves too tight to the scalp
- Braids too tight
- Digging in the scalp with fingernails
- Gelling the hair causing gel buildup in the scalp
- Scratching under finger waves, French rolls, or braids
- Sitting under a overheated dryer too long
- Using high pH shampoos
- Too much sun
- Using hairpins or bobby pins that have lost the rubber tip

Remember to be very scalp conscious. Your elevated awareness within your subconscious mind will not allow you to continue to do things that are harmful to your scalp and that prevent healthy hair growth. It would be useful for you to carry around a small notebook and pen and make a list of things you might be doing to cause damage to your scalp. You want to begin to notice these actions so you can nip them in the bud. Now make a conscious decision not to repeat them. Hold on to your list as a reminder of what you should not do.

**Never chemically treat your hair when your scalp is damaged.**

## YOUR SCALP IS THE FOUNDATION FOR HEALTHY HAIR

You are becoming empowered to achieve your goals of obtaining a healthy scalp as well as healthy hair. You have come to know some things that you may never have thought of before. Your scalp is the foundation, the place from which your hair grows. You have also learned the importance of a healthy scalp to encourage healthy hair growth. You now know that when scalp problems appear, you must never ignore them. You are now empowered to make the positive and correct decisions and choices about scalp care. You will be involved, asking questions and waiting for answers. You will do the necessary research in order to learn more about your scalp and/or any scalp treatments that are prescribed to you.

With this awareness you will always keep in mind that your scalp and hair are connected so your hair care program must address both scalp and hair needs. My seven-week program is both scalp and hair friendly and will not create another problem while solving one. Your seven-week program includes hair and scalp care treatments. It is very

**Remember to be very scalp conscious.**

important that you follow this program completely for seven weeks for best results. Then it is important for you to move on to the hair and scalp maintenance program that will give you better scalp now and for many years to come.

# Your Hair

The next thing to learn about is your hair: how it grows, its layers, and the importance of keeping your hair layers in shape.

## UNDERSTANDING YOUR NATURAL HAIR

Hair is a thread-like appendage of the scalp, and comes in various colors, textures, and types. Healthy hair is beautiful hair, no matter what type of hair it is. There is no such thing as bad hair, all hair is good. When hair is damaged and breaking you will notice that it looks dull and lifeless, and won't hold a style. Damaged hair is sick hair. To keep your hair *beautiful* means to keep your hair *healthy*, and in order to do that you will need a hair program that promotes health. A clear understanding of your own hair will help you succeed in a hair care program.

To be educated about your hair, you need to know the following, and you will learn about all of it in this chapter:

- The layers of hair and their functions
- The difference between hair texture and hair type
- The importance of good elasticity and porosity
- The difference between shedding and breakage
- Hair in its natural state
- Altering your hair
- How there can be multiple types and textures, and different degrees of elasticity and porosity on one head
- How to recognize and be aware of the tools, styling, and combing techniques and products that can damage your hair and scalp

Many black women believe that they must have some type of chemical relaxer in order to manage their hair. That is not true. Kinky hair is very versatile and it is entirely possible to manage your hair while maintaining healthy, natural kinky hair. Many women today are choosing to keep all chemicals out of their hair. Some just want a natural look, while others may feel that wearing their hair natural is a way to be more Afrocentric. My research suggests that the majority of black women who wear their hair chemical free feel they are safe from hair problems. Nevertheless, whether chemically treated or natural, black women are having serious hair and scalp problems.

## HEALTHY HAIR AND SCALP TEST

Just look at your hair and scalp, and answer these questions:
- Does your scalp itch?
- Does your scalp flake?

- Does your hair look dry?
- Do you go more than a week without shampooing?
- Do you see excessive hair in the comb after combing?
- Do you apply chemical relaxer to your hair every six weeks or less?
- Do you use a heated styling tool every time you get ready to go out?
- Do you wish you had hair like someone else's?
- Do you consider a ponytail or a bun a regular hairstyle?
- Do you wear a weave, braids, or a wig in order to let your hair rest from chemicals?

If you said yes to three or more of those questions then you may be headed for serious hair and/or scalp problems.

Knowing how to take care of your hair in its natural state before you make a choice to alter it is a must in order to have healthy hair. You must first understand your hair and how it is made before you can take care of it. The more you learn about your own hair, the more prepared you will be to research any hair problems that may arise and you also will understand what your stylist is saying when he or she is talking to you about hair care.

## Hair Layers and Their Functions

Your hair strand has three parts along its length. The root of your hair strand is located under the scalp, inside the follicle. Some consider the root of the hair as the hair located closest to the scalp, or "new growth"; however, this is incorrect. The hair shaft is the body of your hair strand between the root area and the end. The end, of course, is located at the point of your hair strand farthest from your scalp.

Your hair strand also has three layers of depth: the cuticle, the cortex, and the medulla. The cuticle is the top or primary outer layers on your hair strand. The cuticle has three to ten layers on average. In some cases of extremely coarse hair, there may be as many as thirteen or more cuticle layers on the strand. Healthy cuticle layers are packed tightly together and overlap each other like shingles on a house, each layer varying in size, depending on the texture of that particular strand. I call the cuticle layer the style layer because the condition of this layer dictates how well your hair styles. Healthy cuticle layers will produce an appearance of natural shine and fullness to your hair strands, while damaged cuticle layers will produce a dull, rough, thin, and torn appearance, or in many cases a fly-away or frizzy look. Hair that is extremely fine or damaged may have few or no cuticle layers.

The cortex is the second layer to your hair strand, and lies under the cuticle layers. Color-forming pigments that determine your natural hair color are found in this layer, as well as the bonds that determine whether your hair is kinky or straight. All permanent chemical changes take place in the cortex layer. When a relaxer is applied to your hair, a permanent change from kinky to straight occurs in the cortex layer. If it is a permanent color, it is deposited into the cortex layer of hair. When your natural hair color is changed from dark to light, natural color pigments are being removed from the cortex layer. And when your natural light hair is changed from light to dark, artificial pigments are being deposited in the cortex. If a semi-permanent color rinse is applied to your strands, it is not going to reach your cortex layers as long as your cuticle layers are present. A semi-permanent rinse only deposits pigments within the cuticle layers, which usually last for a few months before eventually fading away. Temporary rinses only stain the top of the cuticle layers and will fade in a few weeks. Keep in mind that the darker the color, the more difficult and damaging it is to remove. And the more frequently you change your hair color, the more you run the risk of damaging both the cuticle and the cortex layers.

The medulla layer is the inner most layer of your hair strand. This protein layer is a hollow canal—the inner circle of your hair strand—and all other layers shape themselves around the medulla.

## HAIR TEXTURE AND TYPE

For years, black women have referred to their hair as a "grade of hair." But I wonder if we really know what "grade of hair" means. After working with women of all ages and looking at my own background, even I was not sure, so I began to ask.

I asked women to define the term "grade of hair," and the answers I received were as follows:

"What kind of hair you have."
"How thick your hair is."
"Good or bad hair."
"Soft or hard."

What grade of hair do you have? Is it a good or bad grade? Fine or thick grade? Soft or hard grade? But what does all this really mean?

**For years, black women have referred to their hair as a "grade of hair." But I wonder if we really know what "grade of hair" means.**

Whatever we mean when we say grade of hair, it doesn't educate us on how to take care of our hair. I have stopped using the term, and I invite you to stop "grading" your own and others' hair as well. Here is real information that will empower your hair.

Your hair strand has texture and a type to it. Hair texture refers to the size of the strand. You may have fine hair (small strands), medium hair (average strands), or coarse hair (large strands).

Fine hair strands are very small in diameter. Fine hair has fewer, smaller cuticle layers. Fine hair strands cannot tolerate excessive pressure or heat from a curling iron, blow-dryer, flat iron, pressing comb, or heat rollers. Fine hair will damage easily because it has fewer protective layers than medium and coarse hair strands. This smaller strand requires the least amount of maintenance products in order to manage.

**I have stopped using the term, and I invite you to stop "grading" your own and others' hair as well.**

Medium hair strands are of average size, have a medium quantity of layers, and can tolerate heat and chemicals better than fine hair. Although this is true, all hair strands burn if the temperature of a heated tool is greater than 150°. So, you must be careful not to overuse heated styling tools or chemicals. I recommend that you avoid pressured heat; instead try a lower, more indirect heat.

Coarse hair strands are the largest of the three, are thicker and are difficult to damage. This explains why many women feel that when their hair becomes damaged, it happens all of a sudden. Because coarse strands are larger, damage first occurs through all the thick layers, wearing them down to thinness. Some women experience their strands thinning and no longer being of coarse texture. Because of the damage, the strands have literally changed in size. I call this a texture change.

All textures—fine, medium, and coarse—can appear within one head of hair. And no matter what size your strand is, it can be damaged. Improper use of heated styling tools and chemicals are the leading cause of hair damage, but even natural hair can be damaged by mishandling and poor care.

Hair type deals with whether your hair is kinky or straight. Straight hair is straight, the end. Kinky hair, on the other hand, comes in many degrees. The first sign of the slightest ripple in straight hair makes it no longer straight, but kinky. This is an important fact because many women who have slight degrees of kinkiness to their hair treat it as if it is straight, and this can cause a lot of hair problems. It is also important to note that on one head you can have many degrees of kinkiness. On any human head you will find multiple textures (size) and types (kinky or straight), and both size and type can vary in degree.

**Hair type deals with whether your hair is kinky or straight. Straight hair is straight, the end. Kinky hair, on the other hand, comes in many degrees.**

## POROSITY AND ELASTICITY

Hair porosity is the hair's ability to absorb moisture and hair products or chemicals. Good porosity within your hair strands is very important because it allows your hair to maintain correct moisture, oil, and protein levels, thus giving healthy hair that radiant look and feel. When porosity becomes poor, your hair will absorb chemicals faster, so it can be overprocessed and damaged easily. It will also be harder for the moisture level in your hair to be balanced. Many women complain that their hair seems to drink up oil and moisturizer. When your hair is over-porous, you will notice that it won't hold a style, it will feel and look dry and brittle, and it will break easily. The reason for this is that the strands' cuticles (top layers) have become worn and thin and are not functioning the way they should.

Hair elasticity is the hair strand's ability to stretch without breaking. It is important to have good elasticity because your hair will need to naturally stretch during combing and handling. Poor elasticity occurs when the hair has been damaged in one or more places. While chemical and heat damage will cause poor elasticity, rough brushing or combing, or other mishandling of your strands, can add to the problem. You can check your hair elasticity by sliding your fingers down a single strand. Before you get to the end, grip the strand close to the scalp and close to the end. Now gently pull. If your hair seems to pop immediately, then your hair elasticity is poor. If your hair gives and stretches without breaking, your hair elasticity is good.

## NATURALLY YOURS: KINKY HAIR

Natural, kinky hair is beautiful, manageable, and lovable. I promise you that to know your hair is to love your hair. Let's come to know our hair in its natural state.

Kinky hair is a type of hair that most blacks have. It is spiral in shape but can vary in degree of kinkiness. In other words, let's say that kinky type hair can be slightly kinky, moderately kinky, or extremely kinky. A strand can be extremely kinky in type without being coarse in texture. This extremely kinky type of strand can be fine in texture, which will mean that this strand is both small and tightly spiraled. Many women mistake extremely kinky hair type for coarse hair texture, and say that their tightly spiraled strands are coarse. This mistake can cause a lot of damage, because those who mistake extreme kinky hair type for coarse hair texture tend to use more heat and chemicals, thinking that is what is needed to manage or control their hair.

You must consider the texture—fine, medium, or coarse—as well as the type   slightly, moderately, or extremely kinky—of your own strands when choosing hairstyles, products, and services. You must also be aware of the variations and combinations of types

**Many women say that kinky hair is fragile and hard to comb, but this is not necessarily true.**

and textures on your head. Be sure to look at, feel, and examine your hair. Learn your true hair texture and hair type so that you will be in control, be able educate others, and be able to stop the misreading of your hair that is causing damage.

Many women say that kinky hair is fragile and hard to comb, but this is not necessarily true. One lady came into my center for a hair analysis; she was wearing her hair natural and seemed to be struggling with her decision to do so. During the hair analysis she sat, listened, and hung on my every word. Afterwards, she looked at me and said, "Before today I really did not think that kinky hair was suppose to be combed." Come on! But during the 1970s we wore curly afros and loved them. We combed our hair then and we can comb and care for our hair now. Did we understand and love our hair more then than we do now? In the 1970s, natural afros were in style, and a large number of blacks—men and women—were wearing them. Now that we have gotten away from natural hair, it seems to be hard to go back. I have found that the reason many women are going natural is not because they want natural hair, but because they are afraid of the damage that chemicals and heat have done. Natural seems the only way to preserve their hair. So, each day they look at that natural hair in the mirror and say, "OK, you wooly stuff, come on and let me see how I can wear you today."

## The Importance of Moisture

Kinky hair type, because its shape tends to have less oil distribution to the strands, can be very dry. The spiral structure of the strand makes it virtually impossible for the hair to receive proper natural moisture and oil lubrication. The oil glands may supply some oil to the scalp, but the oil never makes it down the spiral strands all the way to the ends. The farther away the end is from the scalp (in other words, the longer the hair is), the less likely the oil will reach the hair ends. This makes kinky hair dry in nature.

It is important to moisturize your strands before combing. Look at your kinky natural hair when it is wet. Wet hair has 100 percent moisture level. Now feel the hair, noticing how much softer your natural hair is when wet. Take your fingers and slide them through your hair, and notice that your fingers can slide through more easily when your hair is wet than when your hair is dry. The reason for this is that kinky natural hair type's greatest need is mois-

**Moisturizing will allow you to comb your hair without the tugging or pulling that can result in damage.**

ture. Having a higher moisture level allows each individual natural kinky strand to become more relaxed and not stuck to the next strand. Moisturizing will allow you to comb your hair without the tugging or pulling that can result in damage.

## NATURAL STYLES

I know that not all feel this way, but there are many blacks who go natural and use this as an excuse not to deal with their hair. Let's look at braids, dreadlocks, and other natural hairstyles. These styles may not be combed for weeks or even months, with only oils, fragrances, and braid sprays being applied. Hair must not only be groomed for look, but your scalp and hair must be cleaned and conditioned. If you wear natural styles, you must not forget your scalp and hair. Your scalp and hair will still require of you the appropriate care. I remember one lady who wore dreadlocks, and because of lack of care they began to rot away and fall off. I have also met many women who wear dreadlocks, braids, and other styles and have healthy scalps and healthy hair. If you choose to wear these styles, be sure to do your research. Go to a natural hair care specialist—they are out there, you are just going to have to look for them. And never run to natural style in order to avoid your natural hair. Feed your mind with positive education about natural kinky hair type, and then you will be empowered to care for your natural hair.

Natural, kinky hair, with its multiple degrees of kinkiness all on one head, has special hair care needs that must be addressed in order to maintain its health, just as natural, straight hair does. The problem lies with the way we deal with our hair. So, you must attack the problem and not the hair. Even when kinky hair is pressed or chemically relaxed, underneath, the hair is still kinky type hair and has the same or even greater conditioning requirements. You must clean and condition your hair regularly, at least twice a week. Also, you must supply your hair strands with oil as needed for lubrication, shine, and moisturizer, in order to soften and manage. Many women are confused about whether to use a moisturizer or oil. The best rule to follow is: if your hair feels dry, apply a moisturizer; if your hair looks dry, apply oil; and when the hair both looks and feels dry, apply both. Apply moisture first, then oil to seal and shine. In cases where your scalp is dry, you may apply oil. But remember to notice your climate, look at the shampoo pH, and the other things that you have learned so far and will be learning later in this book.

**Even when kinky hair is pressed or chemically relaxed, underneath, the hair is still kinky type hair and has the same or even greater conditioning requirements.**

## CARING FOR NATURAL KINKY HAIR

The basic requisites for healthy hair are cleanliness and conditioning. I know I'm repeating myself, but you should shampoo and condition the hair at least one or two times a week and more often depending on how active you are. Dirty hair becomes drier and harder to manage, so keeping your hair clean is very important. Condition natural hair once a week with a deep-penetrating protein moisturizer conditioner and daily with oil or moisturizer. Clean hair will enable hair treatments to penetrate the hair shaft, while conditioning will keep your hair strong and manageable.

**How you comb your hair is also very important. Remember never to comb dry hair, as this will only cause more tangles and breakage.**

How you comb your hair is also very important. Keep in mind that for every tangle you carelessly pull out, you are creating two or more new ones. Each new tangle creates a new tear in the hair strand, which will result in hair that will mat, tangle even more, and pull out easily, even with simple combing.

### Combing and removing tangles

First, remember never to comb dry hair, as this will only cause more tangles and breakage. You will need a large-toothed comb, and be sure that the teeth are spaced widely apart. The traditional afro comb may not do. The longer or the more spiral your hair is the larger your comb should be. I have medium to extreme kinky hair type, and I wear a texturizer relaxer which leaves my hair in a wave pattern. I also wear a permanent color in my hair and my hair is shoulder length, so I use a big, plastic, rake-type comb to comb my hair. (You know the old afro rake from the past? Now it comes in hard plastic.) You should purchase your comb from a salon or your local beauty supply. The whole idea is to find a comb that will not pull your hair when you use it. Also, you will need a leave-in conditioner and a moisturizer. Apply the leave-in conditioner followed by the moisturizer directly into the tangled areas, then to your hair ends. Use your fingers to remove all tangles. If you have a problem removing a tangle, then your product may not be getting to the core or middle of the tangle. Apply more leave-in conditioner to tangled areas, then use your forefinger and thumb to massage and press the conditioner into the tangled area, which will release the tangle. Now, using your large-tooth comb and starting at the ends, carefully comb out until you can comb from the hair closest to the scalp.

Now that you have combed the hair, you must not let your hair retangle. Part your hair in sections: four sections for long hair (forehead to nape and ear to ear), and six sections for medium length hair (forehead to nape with three plaits on each side of the center part). For short hair, make small sections over the entire head, then plait the hair.

## PRESSED HAIR

Straightening processes are temporary, as we all know, but the hair may not be natural after pressing. Many women are pressing their hair thinking that this is home base and that there's no way to cause the same damage with a pressing comb as you can cause with relaxer. Unfortunately, that is just not true. If your hair is pressed too often or too much pressure heat is applied, your strands will suffer from heat damage. I call this over-

**If your hair is pressed too often or too much pressure heat is applied, your strands will suffer from heat damage.**

processing with a pressing comb. The way to know if your hair is suffering from this type of heat damage is very simple. Rinse your natural hair with warm water and apply shampoo. Your hair should quickly turn back to its natural kinky state. If you notice that all or part of the strand is still straight, then your hair is overprocessed.

The way to be sure that this does not occur is to change the amount of heat and the frequency with which you use the heat. Every time you use any heated styling tool on your hair, test it with an oven thermometer. The hair cuticle layers start to burn at about 300°, depending on the condition the hair is in. To be safe, I recommend that you stay at 150°. You also need to use only one heating device—in other words, if you press your hair, avoid the curling iron altogether and roll your hair in order to achieve curl and style. You should remember to use a leave-in conditioner and a moisturizer, and let your hair dry naturally or under a table top dryer, never using a blow-dryer.

**To be safe, stay at 150°.**

Avoid pressing the hair with oil because oil heats up faster than a moisturizer and could burn the hair during the pressing process. If you find yourself pressing every few days to "hold your press," remember the first day you press, you burn away maintenance products, and the next day you burn hair. You are headed for over-processed hair that will result in thinning of your hair strands or texture change resulting in hair breakage. So be careful!

## CHEMICALLY TREATED HAIR

Everybody's hair and scalp can be sensitive to chemicals. But your hair and scalp do not have to react negatively if a trained, educated professional applies the chemical process. When a chemical is applied to your hair, your body heat will draw it to your scalp, and if your hair and scalp are damaged, you may suffer a reaction. If you placed a chemical on a healthy area of your arm and let it sit there, it would eventually break down, eat away, and burn the skin and hair on your arm. If you applied it to an area of your arm that has a sore or broken skin, the damage would happen even faster. Your arm would start to burn on contact.

As you learned earlier, your hair and scalp can tolerate chemicals for a short period of time if the scalp and hair are healthy. But you must not take chemicals too lightly. When a chemical is applied to a damaged scalp, first it will itch, then burn. Afterwards your scalp will itch and flake, and can feel tender, tight, and dry as it struggles to heal. The hair itself can become damaged when a chemical is used too often on the hair strands. Damaged hair breaks or frizzes easily, looks dull, dry, and brittle, and does not hold a style. Chemical reactions can be minimized by not applying chemicals to damaged scalp or hair. When a chemical is applied to your hair and it causes your scalp to burn and your hair to break, your scalp and hair have become sensitive.

## PREPARING YOUR HAIR AND SCALP FOR CHEMICALS

Remember, you have control and you know how important it is to care for your scalp. A sensitive scalp and hair come from a damaged scalp and damaged hair. You must avoid all chemicals for a period of time, allowing your scalp to heal and your hair to become stronger. You will also need to allow time for new hair to grow in. As it does, give your hair and

**A sensitive scalp and hair come from a damaged scalp and damaged hair.**

scalp the best care. Clean and condition as needed, avoiding any negative actions. Below I have listed a few things to do to prepare your hair and scalp for chemicals:

- Avoid using shampoos that are of a pH higher than 6.
- Avoid the use of gels on your scalp and hair.
- Shampoo at least every three days, never going longer than seven days.
- Never scratch the scalp or "lift the dandruff."
- Always treat your scalp as skin.
- Limit the amount of heated styling before applying any chemical.
- Sit under the dryer with your conditioning treatments.
- Before your hair is chemically treated, sit under a cold dryer to cool and close scalp pores.
- Apply a scalp base around the hairline and on the scalp area before chemicals (this will depend on the type of chemical).

### The Journey from Kinky to Straight

Let's be realistic about relaxers. You know the risks, but you want it anyway. For some women, the journey from kinky to straight hair begins with a relaxer. Many feel that it is the ultimate way to control or manage kinky hair. But to most, the journey is a neverending cycle of hair and scalp problems. One of my surveys revealed that the average black female experiences major hair loss at least four times in her lifetime while wearing a relaxer.

I feel that women who chemically relax their hair choose to do so simply in order to have style control and more manageability. But so often in their quest to control their hair, they seem to destroy it. The improper use of hair chemical services accounts for more than 50 percent of the hair loss among black women, ranging from chronic hair breakage to baldness. One reason for this problem is that most clients don't take this chemical treatment of their hair seriously enough. As a professional, I am required to pass a state board examination to obtain a license before applying chemicals to my clients' hair. Yet a client can go and buy a relaxer kit over the counter. Don't think just because a relaxer is sold over the counter that it is safe to use at home. When a chemical relaxer is applied to your hair, many changes occur within the hair strand. The chemical travels into the hair going through many cuticle (top) layers of hair until it reaches the cortex (second) layers, then it

**I feel that women who chemically relax their hair choose to do so simply in order to have style control and more manageability.**

breaks delicate bonds and reforms them, allowing your hair to have a more relaxed look.

This is a permanent chemical change that occurs within your hair strands. Therefore, proper analysis and pre-treatment before this service, also proper application, rinsing, shampooing, and conditioning are absolutely necessary in order to ensure that no damage is done to your hair, scalp, and surrounding skin areas. When and if you decide to wear your hair chemically relaxed, a hair and scalp analysis should be done by a licensed, experienced professional who is trained in the application, care, and maintenance of chemically treated hair. Follow these guidelines:

Never allow anyone to relax or color treat your hair unless you have seen their work, and talked to some of their clients, as well as seen and felt their hair.

A relaxer or color should never burn your scalp. If it does, your stylist should stop and treat your scalp until it heals.

Never stay with a stylist if he or she allows your scalp to burn time after time without correcting the problem.

A "retouch" should be applied only on the new growth. Because a relaxer is permanent, overlapping will eventually cause overprocessing and result in hair loss.

Always pay close attention to how your hair is rinsed after a relaxer or permanent color; all chemicals should be rinsed before shampoo is applied.

Never allow a chemical relaxer to be put on your head and left unattended.

Never engage in heavy conversation while your hair is being rinsed. Simply close your eyes and concentrate on your scalp being rinsed. Pay close attention to what your scalp feels like when chemical is around your scalp, and notice to see if that feeling changes after the rinsing is over.

**Concentrate while your hair is being rinsed so you'll feel it if any chemical is left on.**

Never be passive. If your scalp does not feel thoroughly rinsed in some areas or your neck and your crown don't feel as though the water has even touched them, ask to be rinsed again.

After a chemical is rinsed from your hair, the neck strip and towel should be removed and replaced by fresh clean ones, and the neck rest must be sanitized. Then and only then should the shampooing process begin.

A protein and moisturizing, deep penetrating conditioner should be applied to your hair, and you should sit under the dryer for a minimum of fifteen to thirty minutes, in five to ten minute intervals.

### Preventing damage from chemicals

When a chemical relaxer is applied to your hair, many changes occur within the hair strand, very rapidly and automatically. Your cuticle opens and the chemical passes through to the cortex layer. The inner bond of the cortical fibers which hold the hair together begins to break down. Then a separation occurs, and the bonds are formed into a new shape. In the case of a permanent color, the process is slightly different. Although the chemical goes into the cortex layer, it does not change the structure, or shape, of the hair strand. The permanent color will either deposit artificial color pigments or remove natural color pigments from the area of the cortex where your natural pigments lie. As with any chemical, it must be removed and go out the way it came in. In other words, as the chemical leaves the cortex and cuticle layers, the hair starts to rebind and close down and the neutralizing or realigning process begins.

Chemicals cause your hair to go to a pH of 11 to 13, which is very high and dangerous. So, it is very important to bring the hair back to the normal hair and scalp pH. That is why rinsing is so important. Water has a pH of about 7, which is neutral. As water touches your hair and the chemical is rinsed, the pH of your hair begins to change and lower to a more neutral level of 7. Your shampoo must have a pH of 5.5, which is hair pH; this causes the hair to "realign." Most professionals believe that the shampoo will neutralize the chemical, which is not altogether true. Although the shampoo is important, it does not take the place of proper rinsing. If your hair and scalp are not properly rinsed, traces of the chemical will be left on the hair and scalp surface. Water allows the hair strand and scalp to neutralize. Once all of your strands and your scalp have been rinsed thoroughly, then the hair and scalp will be at the pH of water (7). At this point, your technician can be sure that your hair and scalp are ready to be shampooed.

Your technician may instead struggle to remove the relaxer with shampoo. Many believe that they can rinse quickly, thinking that once the shampoo is applied it is supposed to remove the relaxer. But practicing this technique is very dangerous, so I have a high aversion to it. The shampoo should bring the hair back to the correct hair pH, which is 5.5, but it can only do so after the hair has been rinsed properly. Failure to apply these steps in this order will cause problems: your hair will begin to overprocess and then hair loss will occur. Also, your scalp will burn and high level scalp damage will occur.

### Pretreating your hair and scalp

Always pretreat your hair and scalp before a chemical is applied. Although many stylists agree with me, your stylist may not and may frown on this. Some stylists are concerned that pretreating the hair will slow down the chemical process. That is, in fact, the whole idea behind pretreatment. I would never apply a chemical process without pretreating. When a chemical relaxer is applied, even when the most trained and skilled stylist or technician is applying it, overlapping can occur. Continual overlapping will eventually cause overprocessing and damage, so it is better to be safe now, than sorry later. This also is true of permanent color, but one other benefit to pretreating when having a permanent color is that pretreating also helps to equalize the porosity of the hair, allowing the color to process in a more even manner. Because the pretreatment is applied to areas where the relaxer should not be applied, it is OK to slow down the relaxing process. If your stylist

**Always pretreat your hair and scalp before a chemical is applied.**

does not have time to pretreat your hair and scalp, you can do it before you go to the salon. You may be able to save time and money doing it yourself, also.

Pretreating has many benefits and it does not take much time to do. Pretreating your hair and scalp allows your stylist or technician to read your new growth line, because it will be more visible. It also aids in closing the scalp pores on a hot humid day, and helps to lubricate a dry scalp when exposed to dry climates. Pretreatments also equalize the porosity of the hair strands so that certain chemicals can process in a more even manner.

Pretreatments can start up to forty-eight hours before a chemical is applied. How many times have you said, "I didn't do anything to my hair because I knew that I was coming to get my chemical." Many women will wait a week or two to shampoo their hair saying, "My scalp will burn if I shampoo my hair before a chemical." Many women feel that the longer they wait, the better the whole chemical process will go. Actually, the longer you wait, the dirtier your scalp and hair will be. Now, I don't necessarily recommend that you shampoo an hour before your chemical, but forty-eight hours would be just fine. By doing this your hair and scalp will be free from negative buildup, but your scalp pores will not be open to a point that will cause burns. The day of your chemical service, preferably right before you go in, carefully apply oil to your scalp and hairline (not to your hair). Next, lightly apply a leave-in hair vitamin to your strands. When having a relaxer

**Don't wait to shampoo before a chemical process.**

retouch, lightly apply hair vitamins above the demarcation line, the line where your new growth ends and the chemically treated hair begins. Next, carefully spread hair vitamins to the ends of your hair. Remember you are not wetting your hair, only applying enough hair vitamins for the hair to absorb. Be sure to arrive early for your salon appointment. Let your stylist know that you are early and ask your stylist or technician if you can sit under a cold dryer for five minutes before she is ready to apply your chemical. Offer to pay an extra fee, but you can generally expect that there will be no charge. By offering to pay, you will show how important this is to you. Be sure that the products used when pretreating the hair are water-soluble.

### Permanent color and relaxer together

As you know, both permanent relaxer and color cause a chemical change to occur in the cortex layer of the strand. Spacing and timing is crucial in preventing hair breakage. The relaxer goes deeper into the cortex and has a higher pH than the color. The relaxer is, in many ways, a stronger, more forceful chemical. This is not to downplay the dangers of using a permanent color; it can cause a great deal of damage as well. A relaxer, when applied, will travel to the innermost area of the cortex in the breaking-down process. So, when a relaxer is applied right after the hair has been treated with permanent color, the relaxer must go through the area of the cortex where the color change has occurred, causing tremendous damage. In simple terms, your technician must

**Be careful when using permanent color and relaxer together.**

layer your chemical like bricks to prevent damage. A relaxer should be applied first. Then, one week later, your color technician can apply your permanent color.

You must also adjust your maintenance program. When you wear two chemicals, your hair cannot maintain its moisture level, so your hair will dry out and break, feeling like straw. It is important to use a deep penetrating conditioner every two or three days, and to apply a moisturizer each day. Once you notice that your hair is beginning to retain its moisture level or softness, then you can apply moisturizer as needed, but continue your deep conditioning program. Also, make a habit of using a light oil each day before you comb your hair—this will give shine and protection to the cuticle layers.

**When you wear two chemicals, your hair cannot maintain its moisture level.**

Understanding how chemicals affect your hair in no way means that you should use this knowledge to apply your own chemical. All chemical services must and should be applied by a trained and experienced stylist/technician.

## Retouching

Retouching is an area where many women are confused, and chemically relaxing their hair much too often. I have treated women for hair loss and scalp damage who are having relaxer applied as often as every four weeks, or even every two weeks.

Hair strands grow from a healthy human scalp on an average of half an inch every four weeks. Allow your hair to have at least one inch of new growth, ideally one and a half to two inches of new growth, so that the chemical technician has a clear line of demarcation between new hair and chemically treated hair. With a new growth relaxer (retouch), only the new hair, which is not always easily recognized by a professional, should be chemically treated. Overlapping is very difficult to avoid. Applying a relaxer to hair that was previously relaxed will lead to over exposure and overprocessing and, over a period of time, will cause a texture change and then hair loss. A new growth

**Allow at least one inch of new growth before you get a retouch.**

relaxer should be given on an as-needed basis, but never sooner than every eight to ten weeks. Never be in denial about your hair type; always understand that when you choose to straighten your hair, you must be mindful. Remember that underneath that chemically straightened hair there is kinky hair that has been taken through some extreme structural changes.

For years, professionals have cautioned their clients that their hair will break off if they don't get their retouch on time, but that is not necessarily true. You will not lose hair between relaxers if you take control. You have control of your new growth, and if you practice new growth management, your hair will not fall out or break off. It is a must that you learn how to manage the line where your natural new growth ends and your chemically treated hair begins.

I conducted a study to find out why women with kinky hair type struggle with and can't seem to manage their new growth. I needed to understand firsthand and on a day-to-day basis what women go through so that I could come up with answers and create a solution to what seems to be a serious problem. I decided to conduct the study on myself, which would give me the opportunity to experience and gain insight into what happens when our new hair starts to grow in. I wore both a permanent relaxer and permanent hair color; I always waited twelve weeks to relax my new growth; and, I only color-treated my hair twice a year. I managed my new growth without any problems, so I needed to have more of a challenge.

I conducted two studies over approximately sixteen months. The first study lasted seven months, and the second lasted nine months. In the first study, I waited seven months before applying a relaxer to my three and a half inches of new growth, and in the second, I waited nine months before applying relaxer to my four and a half inches of new growth. I learned the most from the seven-month study. As I said, I normally waited twelve weeks between relaxers anyway, so I did not really run into problems until about the fourth month. My hair seemed to mat and tangle more than ever, and no matter what I tried, nothing helped. I would get up in the morning and look at my hair and literally talk to it, saying, "What do you want? I know that I can control you." I was talking to my hair as if it was a person. No matter how carefully I combed my hair, no matter how large the comb that I used, my hair was coming out. I had lost control. I thought to myself, "What are you saying, what are you doing? You can

**You have control of your new growth, and if you practice new growth management, your hair will not fall out or break off.**

control your hair." I stopped and began to focus as I looked at my hair. I realized something very important that I had never thought about before—something that would help me to understand that my hair was not just falling out, I was pulling and thinning my hair out. I began to look at my hair in a different way.

When your hair is chemically treated, your hair actually changes in type from kinky hair type to chemically treated kinky hair type. When your new growth starts to appear, you then have two types of hair: some is chemically treated kinky hair, and some is natural kinky hair. These two very different hair types now share space on each strand, and if you are not careful, one type will dominate.

Now guess which one. You are right—the natural kinky hair will rule. Why? Because there is a line of demarcation, that is, a line of difference. The hair closest to your scalp is what I call baby hair because

**When your new growth starts to appear, you then have two types of hair: some is chemically treated kinky hair, and some is natural kinky hair.**

it has not been in the world long enough to become damaged. It is stronger. It has all its natural spiral shape, all its layers, and its ability to stretch without breaking. There is a line that we must cross to get to the next hair type on the strand, which is chemically treated kinky hair type. Now, this part of the strand has been chemically treated, so the shape is no longer kinky but now straight. This part of the strand is older because it has been on the head longer. It has been through wear and tear, not to mention rough combing and/or brushing and other chemicals, products, and heated styling tools.

Even at best, when the chemically treated kinky hair part of the strand is in optimum condition, new growth management is mandatory. The natural kinky new growth is naturally healthier and stronger. With a new retouch relaxer, all of your hair on the surface of the scalp is straight, so you seem to comb without resistance. Your new growth on average grows to about half an inch in a four week period, and each spiral strand grows from the scalp side by side with the next strand. Because of its spiral shape, the natural kinky hair will begin to intertwine and seemingly lock together. As you comb your hair, you unknowingly pull it, causing stress on the line of difference. The elasticity becomes poor and the hair breaks. As this continues you become more and more frustrated with your hair and may end up causing more damage.

This explains why I was pulling my hair out—my new growth had locked. The longer my hair got, the more my hair would mat and lock. So the solution was in the problem. My hair was not falling out, I was pulling it out because my hair was matting and locking. Once I realized this, I stopped pulling my hair out because I stopped allowing my hair to mat and lock. I started over, right where I was. And I took control, managing my new growth.

I struggled through that first study, but the second one was a breeze. You may ask why I did the second study, and, since it was a breeze, why I ever went back to a relaxer. It was because I wanted to prove that I could manage my new growth without a struggle for as long as I wanted to. I went back to a relaxer because it was my choice to make.

## New Growth Management

Take steps to manage your new growth and you will save your strands. New growth management steps will depend on the degree of kinkiness of your hair. The main thing to remember in new growth management is never to get off track and always to stay on top of things. In other words, the day you say, "I don't need to do anything to my new growth today," will be the day your new growth will take control. When your new growth starts to come in, you must focus your attention and apply all care to new growth first.

> **When your new growth starts to come in, you must focus your attention and apply all care to new growth first.**

Before you shampoo, take your fingers and feel your new growth, then gently caress any tangles away.

Get in the shower, part your hair with your fingers, and allow the force of the very warm water to rinse inside the new growth.

Apply shampoo to your fingers, part your hair with your fingers and gently slide your fingers inside and through your new growth.

Rinse inside your new growth.

Towel blot the inside of the new growth, and on the line of difference.

Apply protein and moisture conditioner inside the new growth in order to stabilize the line of difference.

Allow your fingers to slide through the strands toward the ends.

Place a plastic cap on your head and sit under a warm dryer for ten minutes.

Rinse inside the new growth.

Towel blot, drying inside the new growth.

Lightly apply leave-in hair vitamins to the inside of the new growth, and caress toward the ends of strands.

Follow the above steps, shampooing and conditioning every three days.

## Styling with new growth

You are going to have to adjust your style while you're accommodating your wonderful, healthy new growth. Learn to work with your new growth and not against it. In other words, instead of a straight finished look, try a curlier style. Set your hair on a small to medium roller, depending on the length of your hair. Be sure to limit your dryer time and let your hair dry naturally as much as possible. Try sitting under a warm dryer for a maximum of twenty minutes, then dry naturally. After your hair is dry, apply moisturizer inside the new growth. Each day, feel your new growth and apply a moisturizer there. By putting all the focus on the new growth, the hair is calm—not matting, locking, or tangling—and your scalp is not tender from all that tug of war. You will not lose hair unnecessarily, and you won't feel the need to rush and get a relaxer retouch. You will even begin to enjoy your natural hair.

**You are going to have to adjust your style while you're accommodating your wonderful, healthy new growth. Learn to work with your new growth and not against it.**

# Hair Care Products & Beauty Salons

## HAIR CARE PRODUCTS

With every hair situation, decision, problem, or concern, you must first look and see if this is a basic care, support, or style issue. I have come up with this breakdown because I have found in my studies that you can stay more focused and have more success in dealing with any hair situation if you understand these important issues.

### Basic Care (Shampoo and Conditioner)

How you care for your hair is your foundation, and it basically dictates the health of your hair and scalp. Without a good hair and scalp cleansing and conditioning program, it is like having beautifully decorated walls without a floor. It will only be a matter of time before the walls fall over, so you see where I am headed.

There are two key steps in caring for your hair: cleansing and conditioning. There are three types of products that I recommend: shampoo, conditioner, and leave-in conditioner.

The basic need for healthy scalp and hair is cleanliness. A clean scalp will resist a variety of disorders, while clean hair will enable hair treatments to penetrate the hair shaft. The protein and moisture balance provided by conditioner will give your hair strength, softness, and a healthy appearance of life and body. A leave-in conditioner (what I call hair vitamins) will maintain the physical condition of the cuticle, or outer layers of your hair.

## Support (Oil and Moisturizer)

Support involves shine and softness, and the two products you'll use for these are oil and moisturizer. You'll use these two products to remedy both care and style issues, and you'll be able to use them in conjunction with each other or individually.

An oil lubricates the hair shaft, giving a natural shine and a healthy look even to damaged or dull hair. An oil also aids in the final stage of scalp healing by preventing the flaky dryness that is usually associated with a damaged, dry scalp. If your hair or scalp looks dull and dry, then you should lightly apply oil until you get a nice, natural shine.

Dry hair and a dry scalp both benefit from the use of moisturizers in two ways: first, moisturizers soften dry hair. Second, moisturizers balance and help maintain the moisture level in the hair shaft and scalp. If your hair feels dry or your scalp feels tight and dry, then you should apply moisturizer.

## Style (Set and Hold)

Your choice of style is the image you want to project, or the way you want your hair to look. The basic function of your style is to stop frizzing, puffiness, or limpness, and to improve curl retention and appearance. There are two types of products to use in styling: products that set the style and products that hold the style. I recommend sculptor set and sculptor mist.

A sculptor setting lotion will give you control and versatility in how you style your hair. This type of product works on the cuticle, or outer layers of the hair shaft, to set your hair temporarily in place. A sculptor misting holding spray will block out excess humidity by sealing the cuticle layers, thus holding your style.

## BEAUTY SALONS AND HAIR CARE PROFESSIONALS

In order to have a successful hair care program, you must decide on an attitude towards beauty salons. Some women think of beauty salon visits as social events, a time to talk to other women about things that concern women, while others think of a visit to the beauty salon as a dreaded nightmare. Salon visits are needed for special hair and scalp treatments, all chemical services, and when you want a special cut or style and counsel on

**In order to have a successful hair care program, you must decide on an attitude towards beauty salons.**

home hair and scalp care. I remember that when I got my first job in a beauty salon I was amazed at how long the clients stayed in the salon just to have their hair shampooed and styled. I remember clients coming in and staying an average of six to eight hours. In my opinion that's a *job*. I don't know about you, but if I am going to be there for that amount of time I will be looking for a paycheck.

I did not grow up having my hair done in a salon, so I had never witnessed anything like that before. I thought, "How could anyone just sit there, wait that long, and still pay for the service?" It was not as if they were even being worked on the whole time.

Let me give you an example. One client had an appointment for 9 A.M. She walks in on time and everybody says their good mornings. But by 10 a.m. that client is still sitting; by 11 a.m. that client is still sitting. No one has come up and said anything to her. It was as if she expected the wait and the stylist was not bothered. After about a three hour wait and just when the client was about to walk out, they would shampoo her, then the wait would begin again. It was as if they knew that once they got her head wet she would not leave. Well, add an additional four hours to the time already spent and out came a beautiful hairstyle and a client who seemed to be pleased—but how could she be? Sometimes as I worked I would watch the faces of clients. Some would clearly be very upset and some would seem not to care, as if this was to be expected. Many would bring stacks of paperwork or pack a lunch.

An inconsiderate stylist I once knew might set an appointment for 9 a.m., waltz in herself at 10 a.m., then leave her client under a dryer for an hour or two while she went to the mall to shop. To add insult to injury, she would return and make that poor client wait some more while she showed everybody what she had purchased at the mall.

I know that you are thinking—there is no way on God's green earth that you would sit through an experience like that. But I have interviewed many women who had similar stories and witnessed such behavior firsthand because it happened to them. You must be assertive and stay in control of your salon visits and the way your hair and scalp are cared for while you are in the salon. Many women choose to make weekly or bi-weekly salon visits because they enjoy having someone else shampoo their scalp and hair, and that's OK. What is most important is that you stay in control of all salon visits.

## Managing Your Salon Visits

First, you must decide if and when you need to make salon visits. You also must make your needs known. Let your stylist know that your time is important. You should be understanding of some wait, but all concerned must be considerate of each others' time.

1. Be on time for your appointments.

2. If for any reason you will be late, call and ask if you need to reschedule.

3. Always give twenty-four hours, or better yet, forty-eight hours notice if you are going to miss an appointment unless it is an emergency, and even then send an apology card in the mail with an offer to pay for the missed service.

4. Always communicate your likes and dislikes.

Behaving according to the above list will communicate to your stylist by your actions that you are a considerate person and you will not tolerate any inconsiderate actions on his or her part.

### Salon dependency

Be aware never to become "salon dependent." It is and should always be your choice when you make salon visits; however, if you choose to make weekly salon visits, be sure it is truly your desire to do so and it is *not* because you cannot manage your own hair. You should never say

**Never become salon dependent.**

that you can't do your own hair. Remember, you have the power and you can be in control, learning how to style and manage your own hair and only visiting your salon as needed. You will have a new feeling of freedom if you learn how to care for and style your hair between salon visits. With this book you will become educated on proper scalp and hair care. You will become *educated* so you will not cross the line and do things to your hair that should be done in a salon by professionals. You will make salon visits on an as-needed basis, and you will be empowered to be in control of your beauty salon visits, and to make your needs clear to your hair care professional.

### Choosing a Hair Care Professional

Your hair care professional makes a living from services rendered. It is up to you to insist that he or she serves you in the proper way. You may have more than one hair care professional. There are many licensed professionals in beauty salons who have different areas of expertise.

Unfortunately, most licensed hair professionals will say that they can do it all. You may go to one salon because you are having hair problems, and ask if they can stop your hair problems, and they will say, "Sure, I can do whatever you need." That person may have a license, but if they have not taken the time to do the research and become trained in the area of hair and scalp problems, then you may end up with more problems than before you walked in their door. One of the reasons many who are licensed to do hair will

**Your hair care professional makes a living from services rendered. It is up to you to insist that he or she serves you in the proper way.**

say, "I can do it all," is because the cosmetology industry has done a poor job in the area of specializing individuals that are licensed in hair. In other words, if you go to beauty school to obtain a cosmetology license, then you are allowed to do it all. To tell you the truth, when I received my cosmetology license I really felt like a jack of all trades and a master of none. I know that there are many professionals who will frown and not be pleased with what I am saying, but many will agree with me. Now, I love this industry and had one of the best cosmetology teachers around, but I had to research, come up with theories, then conduct studies to prove my theories in many areas. I felt that many of these areas should have been a part of the core curriculum, and they simply were not.

I mention all of this in order to say to you, be aware. When you are choosing a stylist, it is up to you to be assertive and take the time to find the correct hair and scalp care professional. Remember this is your hair and you are paying your stylist to serve you. It is worth it to do the extra research necessary.

Friends, family, coworkers, and even people you see in the mall or at the grocery store can help you find the right hair care professional. If you notice someone who has healthy hair, first compliment her on her hair. When you compliment someone, they usually will be willing to give you any information. Ask a few simple questions. Number one, are you happy with your hair care professional? If someone lists more than two things they dislike about their hair professional, then you might want to pass. If the answers are positive, take it from there. Ask for the name and phone number of the salon, and for the professional's name.

Be resourceful. Another way to find a hair care professional is to check the phone book. I know you may not know them, but when you call a salon, most will be happy to gain a new client and will be glad to answer your questions about their stylists and the salon's services. Ask for an appointment for a consultation with that professional. Salons and professionals are interested in building and keeping a clientele and should allow this appointment. Take with you a list of your hair and scalp care needs and concerns. Be assertive. Ask complete questions and wait for complete answers. Make your choice based on how well the consultation goes. It may take consultation appointments with many salons before you find the right one, so be patient. Remember, the answer is in every question and the solution is in every problem.

### Be assertive

Here are three golden rules to keep in mind when you visit a beauty salon.

1.  Never be *passive* while in a salon or when talking to your hair and scalp care professional.
2.  Never be *aggressive*.
3.  Always be *assertive*.

Be fully aware of what is being done to and used on your hair and scalp. Ask questions. Decide what you want from your hair care professional and salon. Make a list of things that you *will* and *will not* accept in a salon visit and from a hair professional. You will be able to choose a hair professional from the list of things you will and will not accept. For example, if you are wearing natural hair, you need a professional who is educated in the care and maintenance of natural hair. The same applies if you are using a relaxer, color, or would like a special cut, style, or whatever. The important thing is to let your educated subconscious mind be your guide, and then start your search.

| Will Accept | Will Not Accept |
| --- | --- |
| A true professional | Someone with an arrogant or careless attitude |
| A clean salon | A dirty salon |
| Thorough shampooing | An itchy and flaky scalp after a shampoo |
| Proper conditioning | Too little conditioner applied |
| A neck rest that is sanitized | A dirty neck rest |
| A clean towel after chemicals | A wet or soiled towel |

| Will Accept | Will Not Accept |
|---|---|
| Hair talk and limited casual talk | Gossip and other negative talk |
| Relaxing music | Loud, harsh, or insulting music |
| My hair being handled with care | My hair carelessly combed and pulled |
| Chemicals done properly | Overlapping, overprocessing, improperly applied chemicals |
| Hairstyled with care | Hair overheated, stressed, or damaged into a style |
| A reasonable amount of dryer time | Excessive time under the dryer and dried out hair and scalp |
| Timely services | Long waits before services and overbooking |
| A reasonable amount of time in the salon | Four, five, six, and seven hour salon visits |
| Someone educated about my hair needs | Someone not specializing in my hair needs |
| Someone who is willing to listen | Someone who ignores me or treats me as if I am stupid |
| Someone who cares | Someone only interested in making money |

Make this list your own, and feel free to add your own acceptable and unacceptable terms. Even if it takes you some time and energy to locate the right salon and hair care professional, it will be worth the investment.

# Conclusion

Once you have completed this program and improved your hair, you will want to maintain the health of your hair and prevent problems from returning. Many of you have extremely damaged hair that will require continual care and consideration as your healthy new hair grows in. Be careful to baby your reconditioned hair because, even though it will be stronger than before, nothing can make your old hair as strong as the new hair that is growing in behind it. You must always keep a healthy hair and scalp regimen. You can use what this book teaches you to protect, preserve, and nurture your hair and scalp now and in the years to come.

This program can be repeated in detail as many times as you like, but you may decide, as many have, to turn this program into a lifetime commitment to nurturing your scalp and hair. Just remember that in order to maintain a better head of hair, you first need to maintain a healthy mind and a positive attitude toward yourself and your hair.

# Index

# About the Author

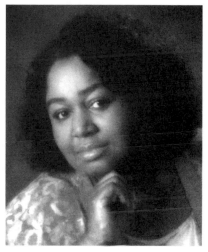

*Photograph by: Rebecca S. Tierce*

Lisa Akbari is a hair care pioneer. For most of her life she has worked in the hair care industry. She became a licensed cosmetologist in 1977. By the age of twenty-one she had opened her first salon. As a stylist, Mrs. Akbari has always maintained a large clientele and worked on many hair teams and as a platform artist. As an educator she has trained hundreds of stylists and hair care professionals on how to create hairstyles without sacrificing the health of their clients' scalp and hair. Mrs. Akbari owns and operates the Hair Nutrition Research Center in Memphis, Tennessee. Through research and studies, she has discovered several hair and scalp disorders including Short Hair Syndrome and Follicular Epidermis Alopecia. She has successfully created a hair care product line engineered specifically to the needs of African Americans. Mrs. Akbari has a degree in trichology, the study of hair and its disorders, and continues to further her education. She is the author of *The Journey from Kinky to Straight (and All Its Pit Stops)*, and has written countless workbooks and manuals, lead seminars, and recorded videotapes and audiocassettes. Mrs. Akbari is married to Dr. Hooshang Akbari, and has twin daughters, Raumesh and Raumina. She lives in Memphis, Tennessee.